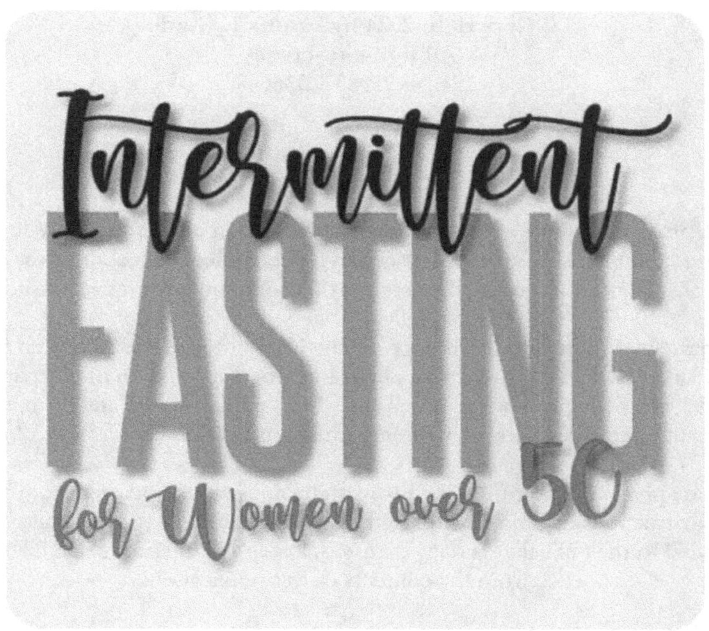

THE ULTIMATE GUIDE TO BOOST METABOLISM, SHED POUNDS, AND REVITALIZE YOUR LIFE WITH EASY STEPS

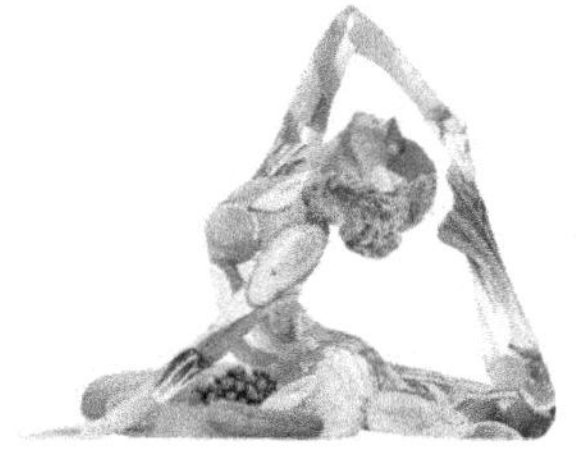

BY

EMMA J. GUIDE

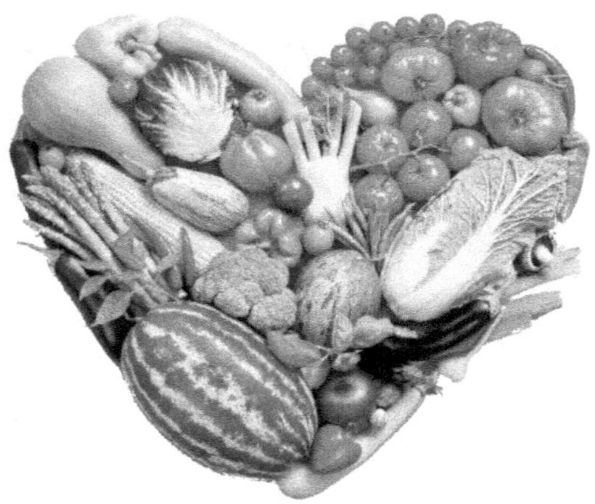

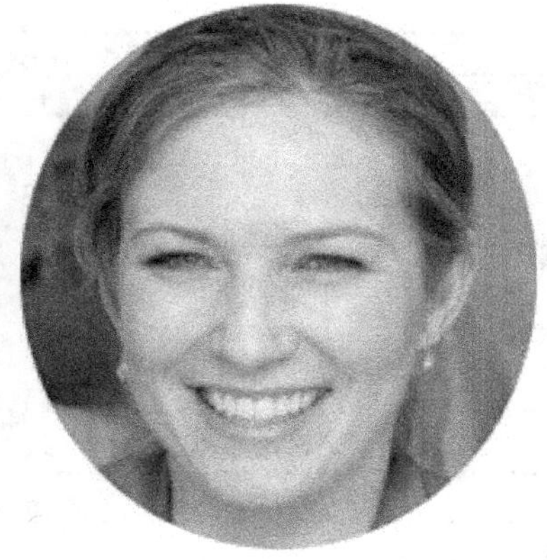

Emma J. Guide's journey into the realm of health and wellness began not in a classroom, but during personal struggle and discovery. Facing the challenges of managing her own health after turning 50, Emma found herself navigating through the overwhelming sea of dietary advice, fitness trends, and health fads. It was during this period of trial and error that she stumbled upon the transformative practice of Intermittent Fasting (IF).

Unlike many who preach from a pedestal of lifelong fitness fanaticism or nutritional science degrees, Emma's expertise is drawn from her lived experience and the palpable empathy she has for others facing similar struggles. Her transition wasn't just about losing weight or looking younger; it was a profound journey toward reclaiming her health, vitality, and zest for life. This transformation was so impactful that Emma felt compelled to share her discoveries with the world.

Armed with a passion for helping others and an insatiable desire for knowledge, Emma dedicated years to studying the intricacies of nutrition, the science of aging, and the psychological aspects of dieting and lifestyle changes. But her approach has always been one of relatability and practicality. Emma understands that the most profound shifts come from sustainable, informed changes rather than quick fixes.

Emma's work, therefore, extends beyond the conventional. She doesn't just share a diet plan; she offers a blueprint for a lifestyle transformation. Through her guidance, countless individuals, especially women over 50, have found a path to improved health, energy, and a renewed sense of self. Her methods aren't just about fasting; they're about feeding the soul with mindfulness, joy, and a deep connection to one's body.

Today, Emma continues to inspire with her story, not as a distant expert, but as a friend who walks the path of wellness alongside you. Her narrative is not found in the digital footprints of social media but in the lives of those she's touched, in the vibrant health and happiness of her community, and in the quiet moments of gratitude from those who've found their way back to themselves through her guidance.

☆ **Here Is the First Tip: <u>Start Now</u>!**
I Can Already Feel Your Satisfaction. It's time to decide and plan a healthier life for yourself and your family. Then, with a straightforward purchase that you can set up in your kitchen, you can begin cooking delicious meals suitable for your body and soul.

So, What Are You Waiting For? It's Time for You to Take Charge!

<u>WE'D LOVE TO HEAR YOUR THOUGHTS!</u>

Dear Reader,

Firstly, we want to extend our heartfelt thanks to you for embarking on this journey with "***Intermittent Fasting for Women Over 50***."
We hope it has illuminated a path toward understanding your body better and has empowered you with tools to achieve your health and wellness goals.

If you've found any part of this book helpful, enlightening, or inspiring, we kindly invite you to share your experience. **Your honest review on Amazon.com** would not only be invaluable to us but also to others just like you, searching for a guide that speaks to their unique challenges and aspirations.

Leaving a review is simple, yet it can make a profound difference. It helps us continue to improve and, more importantly, supports a community of individuals on similar paths, offering them insight and encouragement when they need it most.

To leave a review, just visit our book's page on Amazon.com, scroll to the **'Customer Reviews'** section, and click '*Write a Customer Review*.' Whether it's a few words or a few paragraphs, your feedback is greatly appreciated and eagerly awaited.

Thank you again for your support and for being a valued part of our community.
Together, we can make the journey toward health and happiness not just a possibility, but a reality.

Warmest regards,
Emma J. Guide

TABLE OF CONTENT

5 Exclusive Bonuses Just For You!

Congratulations on taking the first step towards a healthier, more vibrant life with **"Intermittent Fasting for Women Over 50**." As a token of our appreciation and to further support you on this journey, we've prepared some exclusive bonuses.

Here's What Awaits You:

⇒ An enlightening **Q&A** answering the most common questions and offering clarity and confidence as you embark on this path.

⇒ A **Weekly Shopping List** to simplify your grocery shopping experience.

⇒ A **Quick Guide to Smart Food Card** to empower you with knowledge for making the best food selections.

⇒ A **2-Weekly Exercise Plan** designed to complement your intermittent fasting journey and enhance your results.

⇒ A detailed **Meal Planning Journal** to help you organize and optimize your eating windows.

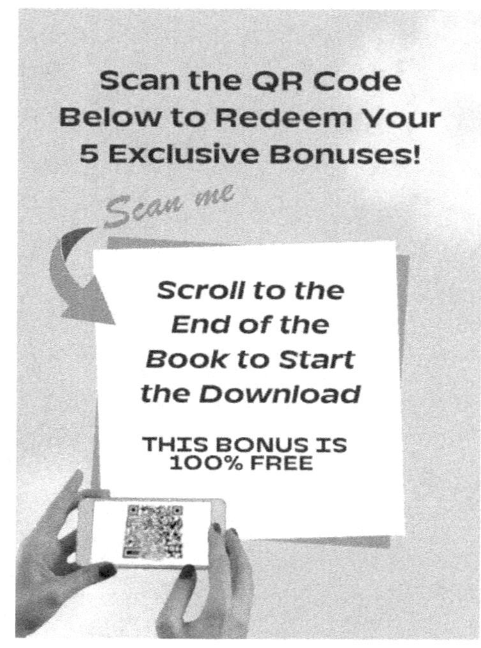

Access Your Bonuses Now. To access these valuable resources, simply scan the QR codes below with your smartphone. Each code will take you directly to one of your exclusive bonuses, ready for download and immediate use.

Let's Get Started! These bonuses have been crafted to enhance your intermittent fasting experience, providing you with tools and knowledge for a successful journey. Scan, download, and start enjoying your bonuses today!

"The promise of a transformed life has never been more attainable."

Intermittent Fasting (IF) ranks among the world's most popular health and fitness trends, embraced by many for its potential to aid in weight loss, enhance health, and simplify lifestyles. Numerous studies highlight its significant impacts on both the body and brain, suggesting it might even boost longevity. IF is characterized by alternating periods of eating and fasting, prescribing not what foods to eat but rather when to consume them. This approach, more accurately described as an eating pattern than a diet, offers a unique regimen for daily consumption. Intermittent Fasting involves alternating between fasting and eating on a regular schedule. Research has demonstrated its effectiveness in aiding weight loss and potentially preventing or even reversing disease.

So, how does one begin, and is it safe?

Two prevalent IF methods include daily sixteen-hour fasts or fasting for an entire day twice a week. Unlike many diets that focus on what to eat, IF emphasizes when you eat. It restricts food intake to specific times of the day, aiding in weight loss. Additionally, empirical research supports various health benefits of this practice. Our ancestors, who were hunters and gatherers before the advent of agriculture, thrived on similar fasting intervals due to the sporadic nature of their food sources. Consultation with a healthcare provider before starting IF is advisable. Once you have approval, the actual practice is straightforward. One common approach is the 16/8 method, restricting daily eating to a 6 to 8-hour window, thereby fasting for the remaining 16 to 18 hours. Another method, the 5:2 diet, involves normal eating five days a week and consuming just one 500–600 calorie meal on the other two days. For example, you might normally eat every day except Mondays and Thursdays, which are designated as your one-meal days. Extending fasting periods to 24, 36, 48, and even 72 hours without food can be less beneficial and potentially risky.

Extended periods without eating may prompt your body to begin storing fat in response to the absence of food. Experts report that adjusting to Intermittent Fasting can take two to four weeks, during which you might experience hunger or irritability. However, those who persist through the adjustment period often find the strategy more manageable overtime, experiencing benefits like weight loss, consistent energy, and decreased cravings. While IF offers numerous advantages, it's crucial to recognize that it may not suit everyone, particularly women. This book delves into the benefits and potential drawbacks of IF for women, providing guidance on how to navigate this dietary approach effectively. Intermittent Fasting has soared in popularity in recent years, touted for its ability to facilitate weight loss, fat reduction, lower blood pressure, and decrease diabetes risk. With these purported benefits, it's no wonder many, especially women, are curious about IF.

Historically, fasting was practiced for religious reasons, but today, more people are exploring IF for its potential health benefits. Although some evidence supports these claims, it's important to note that IF can impact women's hormones, fertility, and bone health differently. The diet's restrictive nature may also contribute to disordered eating patterns. In this book, we explore Intermittent Fasting comprehensively—what it entails, its benefits, potential risks, and how to implement it thoughtfully. Intermittent Fasting's growing popularity stems from its simplicity and the significant health benefits it offers, such as weight loss and improved metabolic health. Unlike other diets that restrict what to eat, IF introduces fasting as a part of your daily routine, potentially helping you consume fewer calories, lose weight, and reduce the risk of chronic diseases. However, evidence suggests that IF might affect women differently than men, necessitating a tailored approach. This book aims to provide a comprehensive guide for women interested in IF, offering a step-by-step approach to fasting that considers the unique needs of women. Remember, there is no one-size-fits-all solution to dieting, including IF. Women might benefit from a more flexible approach to fasting, incorporating shorter fasting periods, fewer fasting days, or consuming a limited number of calories on fasting days.

When distinguishing fact from fiction about IF, being well-informed allows for correct fasting practices, increasing the likelihood of experiencing the benefits such as weight loss and consistent energy that have made IF popular. Unfortunately, misinformation abounds. You may have heard that fasting slows metabolism, leads to muscle loss, or that you shouldn't drink liquids while fasting. However, these theories are often based on speculation rather than evidence. This book will debunk major intermittent fasting myths, enabling you to make informed decisions about incorporating IF into your health regimen. Everyone who starts intermittent fasting typically has a goal in mind—be it for weight loss, improved health, or enhanced metabolic health. Identifying your overall objective can help determine the most suitable fasting method and how to adjust your calorie and nutrient intake. Fasting harks back to early humans who often went hours or days without eating due to scarce resources. Our bodies have adapted to survive—and thrive—on fewer meals, a principle that intermittent fasting seeks to emulate. Intermittent Fasting for nutritional reasons has shown to be incredibly effective for weight loss.

Indeed, most individuals try IF to shed pounds, supported by studies that link fasting to significant reductions in body weight and visceral fat, compared to more traditional calorie-restriction diets. Additionally, fasting has been recognized for its role in managing metabolic syndrome and diabetes, increasing lifespan, protecting neural functions, and showing promise in treating certain gastrointestinal diseases.

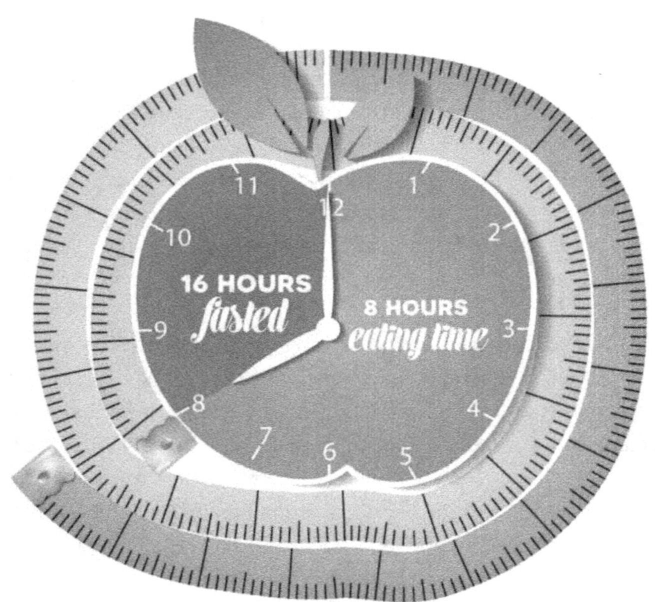

Chapter 1.
BASICS OF INTERMITTENT FASTING

Intermittent Fasting (IF) has become one of the most popular health and fitness trends worldwide. It is celebrated for its ability to help individuals lose weight, improve overall health, and simplify dietary habits. Research has demonstrated significant benefits of IF on both brain and body functions, and it is even suggested to potentially enhance longevity. Historically, our ancestors thrived on intermittent eating patterns. Before the advent of agriculture, humans were hunters and gatherers, enduring long periods without food which required significant physical effort. This lifestyle contributed to maintaining a healthier weight—a stark contrast to modern habits where technology and convenience allow constant access to food and entertainment, contributing to a sedentary lifestyle. This shift has led to an increase in metabolic diseases such as obesity, type 2 diabetes, and heart failure. Current studies have shown that adopting intermittent fasting can help reverse these trends by mimicking the natural eating rhythms of our ancestors.

1.1 WHAT IS ACTUALLY INTERMITTENT FASTING?

Intermittent Fasting involves alternating between periods of eating and fasting. Unlike traditional diets that specify which foods to eat, IF focuses on when to eat. This approach is more about timing rather than dietary restrictions, making it not just a diet, but a lifestyle change. IF schedules vary, with some of the most common being 16-hour daily fasts or 24-hour fasts twice a week. Research supports the effectiveness of IF in promoting weight loss and improving health markers such as blood pressure, cholesterol, and blood sugar levels. However, it is essential to approach IF with care, as it requires significant lifestyle changes and can be challenging to adapt to.

Despite these challenges, an increasing body of evidence supports the strategic timing of fasts as a practical and reliable approach to managing weight and preventing diabetes. Intermittent fasting is deeply rooted in human history, not just as a survival mechanism but also for religious and spiritual reasons across various cultures including Christianity, Islam, Buddhism, and Judaism. Today, IF offers a return to this more natural eating pattern, which is believed to be more in sync with our physiological needs than frequent meals throughout the day.

THE BACKSTORY OF IF

Intermittent Fasting (IF) has roots that trace back long before it gained mainstream popularity in 2012. The premise behind IF is straightforward yet scientifically profound. During fasting, enzymes break down food into molecules like glucose, which our bodies use for energy. Any excess glucose is stored as fat. IF capitalizes on this by varying the timing of meals to reduce insulin levels, which in turn helps the body to use stored fat as energy. This process not only aids in weight loss but also improves metabolic health.

THE SCIENCE OF TIMING IN IF

The effectiveness of IF isn't just about what or how much you eat but when you eat. Research indicates that aligning our mealtimes with our body's natural circadian rhythms, which suggest eating during daylight hours and fasting at night, can enhance health outcomes. Studies involving time-restricted eating show that compressing eating windows can lead to significant health benefits such as lower blood sugar levels, improved insulin sensitivity, and reduced blood pressure.

PRACTICAL INSIGHTS AND RESEARCH FINDINGS

Modern research into IF has explored various fasting schedules. One notable study on "early time-restricted eating" placed all meals within an eight-hour window (7 a.m. to 3 p.m.) and compared it to a more extended twelve-hour eating period. Results indicated no weight gain or loss in either group, but those with the restricted eating window experienced notable improvements in health markers, including appetite control, which was not driven by hunger.

WHY CHANGING MEAL TIMING IS EFFECTIVE

Adjusting meal timing can influence a wide range of biological functions. Transitioning from eating to fasting states triggers important cellular responses beyond simply burning calories. Recent in-depth analyses of IF show that these changes enhance digestion, reduce inflammation—which can alleviate conditions like arthritis—and bolster cellular cleanup, which can decrease cancer risk and boost brain health.

IS INTERMITTENT FASTING SUITABLE FOR EVERYONE?

While the benefits of IF, such as improved metabolic profiles and potential weight loss, are compelling, it's not ideal for everyone. Medical advice is crucial, especially for individuals with conditions like diabetes, or those who are pregnant, breastfeeding, or have a history of eating disorders. IF should be customized to fit individual health needs and lifestyles, ensuring it is a sustainable part of a healthy diet and exercise routine.

RECOMMENDATIONS FOR ADOPTING IF

For optimal health outcomes:

- Avoid sugars and processed grains. Opt for a balanced, plant-based Mediterranean diet rich in fruits, vegetables, legumes, whole grains, lean proteins, and healthy fats.

- Encourage fat burning by fasting between meals—avoid snacking or eating late at night.
- Consider trying simple forms of IF like eating your meals between 7 a.m. and 3 p.m., or from 10 a.m. to 6 p.m., and fasting overnight.
- Maintain active during the day to enhance muscle tone and overall energy levels.

THE PROMISE OF INTERMITTENT FASTING

Why opt for daily calorie reduction when intermittent fasting offers a way to manage weight by modifying when you eat?

This approach allows for normal eating on some days while significantly reducing intake on others, aligning with natural body rhythms, and showing promising health benefits. Whether it's fasting every other day or following a 5:2 diet, IF provides a flexible framework that can be adapted to meet diverse dietary needs and preferences, proving effective in both clinical trials and real-world applications.

1.2 GETTING STARTED

You've already undergone a lot of extended Fasting in your life. If you've ever eaten dinner but slept late the next day and didn't feed before noon, you've fasted for 16 hours or more. This is how some people feed naturally. In the morning, they do not feel hungry. Some people still consider the 16/8 approach to be the most straightforward and long-lasting method for intermittent Fasting; you may want to start there. If you like fasting and feel healthy while doing so, you might progress to more extreme fasts such as 24-hour fasts 1 to 2 times a week (Eat-Stop-Eat) or just consuming 500–600 calories 1 to 2 days a week (5:2 diet). Another choice is to quickly fast anytime it is convenient; simply miss meals when you aren't hungry or don't have time to prepare from time to time. To reap at least any of the rewards, you don't need to implement a formal intermittent fasting schedule. Experiment with various methods before you discover one that you like and work into your routine. It's best to begin with the 16/8 approach and work your way up to longer fasts later. It's crucial to try out different methods before you discover one that fits you.

SHOULD YOU TRY IT?

Anyone does not need to practice Intermittent Fasting. It's just one of the lifestyle interventions that can enable you to lead a healthier existence. The most important items to remember are to consume healthy food, exercise regularly, and have adequate sleep. However, if you don't like the idea, you should quickly dismiss this and go about your day. There is no such concept as a one-size-fits-everyone diet whenever it comes to nutrition. You can choose a routine that you can sustain overtime. Fasting is beneficial to a small number of people, although it is not beneficial to others. You would find out which group you belong to only by trying things out.

Fasting may be an effective strategy for losing weight and improving your fitness if you like it and believe it to be a sustainable form of eating.

HOW DOES IT AFFECT YOUR CELLS AND HORMONES?

So many things occur in your body on a cellular and molecular basis as you are hard. To make retained body fat more available, the body changes hormone levels, for example. Essential repair mechanisms and gene expression changes are often initiated by your cells. When you are hard, your body goes through a few adjustments.

HUMAN GROWTH HORMONE (HGH)

Development hormone levels skyrocket, often by as many as 5-fold. This has many advantages, including weight loss and muscle gain.

- **Insulin:** Insulin response increases, and insulin levels decrease significantly. Lower insulin levels allow stored body fat more available.
- **Cellular repair:** When you are fasting, your cells begin to rebuild themselves. Autophagy is a process in which cells ingest and destroy old and inactive proteins that have accumulated within them.
- **Gene expression:** Changes in the role of genes linked to survival and disease resistance have been discovered. Intermittent Fasting's health advantages are due to improvements in hormone levels, cell structure, and gene expression. Human growth hormone levels increase while insulin levels fall as you fast. Cells in your body also regulate gene expression and activate critical cellular repair processes.

1.3 INTERMITTENT FASTING PLANS

Before beginning intermittent Fasting, make sure to see the doctor. The actual procedure is easy if you have his or her permission. You may use a regular solution, which limits regular eating to a 6 to 8-hour cycle. For example, you might try 16/8 fasting, which involves eating for 8 hours, or fasting for sixteen. Williams is a proponent of the regular regimen: She believes many people find it easier to stay with this routine for the long run. Another method, known as the 5:2 solution, entails eating five times a week. You only eat one 500–600 calorie meal on the remaining two days. For instance, suppose you decided to normally eat any day of the week, excluding Mondays and Thursdays, which are your one-meal days. Fasting over longer amounts of time, such as 24, 36, 48, and 72 hours, is not always beneficial and may be risky. Traveling too long without eating can cause your body to begin storing fat as a response to the lack of food. According to expert reports, it will take two to four weeks for the body to adjust to Intermittent Fasting. When you're getting used to all the new schedules, you may feel hungry or irritable. According to experts, test participants who make it past the transition process are more likely to adhere to the strategy, and they feel stronger.

Water and zero-calorie drinks, including black coffee or tea, are allowed on days that you aren't consuming. And "regularly eating" during your cycles does not imply "going insane." If you fill your meals with high-calorie fast food, super-sized fried foods, and desserts, you're not going to drop weight or get healthy. However, most people choose intermittent Fasting because it helps them to consume and appreciate a variety of foods. We expect people to be aware of their surroundings and enjoy consuming healthy, nutritious food. Eating with each other and enjoying the mealtime moment, she continues, adds pleasure, and promotes good health. Whether you're attempting intermittent Fasting or not, most medical authorities consider the Mediterranean Diet to be a healthy blueprint for what to consume. When you want complex, unrefined carbs like whole grains, green vegetables, healthy fats, and lean protein, you can't go wrong.

1.4 INTERMITTENT FASTING BENEFIT

Intermittent Fasting does more than burn fat, according to research. Changes in this metabolic switch influence the body and the brain. One of the studies that were conducted revealed information regarding a variety of health advantages linked to the discipline. A healthy lifestyle, a leaner frame, and a stronger mind are among them. Intermittent Fasting causes numerous changes in the body that defend tissues from chronic diseases, including type 2 diabetes, coronary failure, age-related neurodegenerative conditions, inflammatory bowel disease, and several cancers. Whenever it comes to weight reduction, there are two theories as to why IF might be successful. First is that Fasting creates a net calorie deficiency, which causes you to lose weight. Another definition is more complicated: this technique might avoid what is known as the "plateau phenomenon." After six years, the researchers found that, after the initial remarkable weight loss, the participants had recovered most of their weight and that their metabolic rates had slowed, resulting in them burning even fewer calories than would have been anticipated.

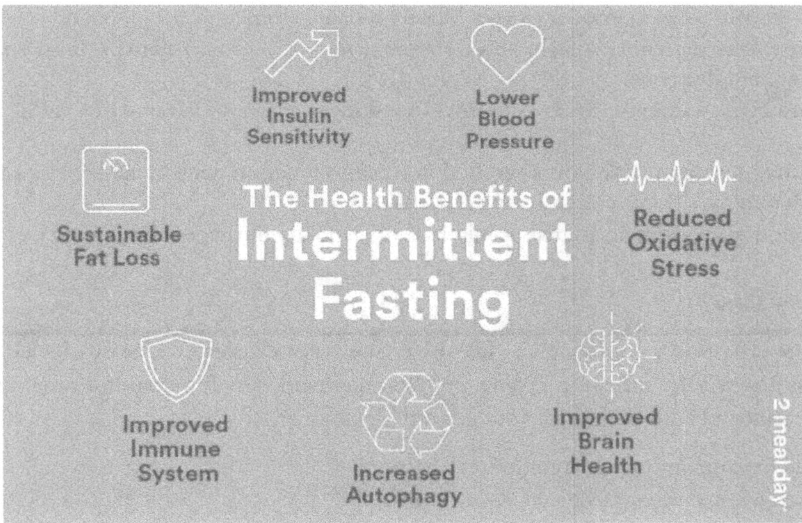

While a study on the efficacy and safety of IF is required, one of its touted advantages is that it may avoid metabolic sputtering. Often individuals who want to lose weight through diet and exercise wind up falling off the wagon and gaining weight. Hormones that stimulate weight gain, such as appetite hormones, are activated, and it's assumed that intermittent Fasting (IF) could help avoid this metabolic adaptation.

Normal eating patterns in IF "trick" the body into dropping weight until it reaches a plateau. No, does it help you lose weight? Proponents of the proposal have agreed in a resounding yes based on anecdotal proof. It does fit with anyone who will stick to IF. However, proponents of the method argue that it is about far more than just getting a lean body. Clients are told that they can improve their insulin sensitivity (lowering their risk of type 2 diabetes), reduce inflammation, and "boost survival by improving the quality of your mitochondria," according to a specialist nutritionist (cell powerhouses). Over eight weeks of IF, obese individuals shed an average of 12 pounds while simultaneously lowering their overall cholesterol, "bad" LDL cholesterol, and systolic blood pressure, according to one small report. Research showed that while 12 weeks of IF had little effect on cholesterol levels, it did result in weight loss and a reduction in systolic blood pressure. A study investigated 11 IF trials of overweight or obese people that lasted at least eight weeks. Nine of those experiments found that an IF regimen was almost as successful at having people shed weight and body fat as conventional dieting when opposed to cutting calories every day.

However, it's worth noting that researching the human lifespan is much more complex than studying weight loss. That's why, as a report suggested, most of the research that says IF encourages a longer life span has been conducted in species, including fruit flies. Another study found that the physiological benefit of Intermittent Fasting is that it puts your body into a condition of ketosis (the keto diet's metabolic state), where fat is burned instead of carbohydrates for energy. The concept that ketones can activate the body's own repair mechanism, eventually defending against disease and aging, goes beyond the weight-loss impact, according to the researchers. It's also crucial to keep the hopes in check. Because a lot of testing is focused on animals, it's more challenging to adopt the findings to people who are obviously free-thinking and must contend with the consequences of lifestyle problems such as job pressures, insane schedules, emotional eating, and cravings, to name a couple, all of which may impair one's desire to adhere to a particular diet. While it seems to be promising, it is "no more successful than any other eating plan."

Here are a few of the proposed IF advantages:

- **Boost weight loss:** According to a study, most of the evidence on IF has backed its contribution to weight reduction, with evidence indicating that it might result in a loss of 5 to 9.9% of body weight. Alternate-day Fasting could result in greater fat loss than time-restricted feeding, according to a 2018 report, but alternative Fasting may be more difficult to maintain than time-restricted eating. Finally, further study is required to see if this IF will lead to actual, long-term weight loss.
- **Lengthen life;** According to one report, calorie restriction can help to slow down the aging process. However, the research was conducted on primates, and the results are yet to be replicated in humans.
- **Reduce insulin resistance;** According to a report conducted in 2014, insulin resistance is a symptom of type 2 diabetes, and becoming overweight raises the risk of insulin resistance. According to a report published in 2019, you can assist with insulin tolerance by lowering total calorie consumption.
- **Improve metabolic parameters;** What we do know is that many of those metabolic parameters change in response to weight loss. You'll see less abdominal (belly) fat, lower fasting blood sugars, lower triglycerides, lower blood sugar, and so on, no matter if you drop weight. According to experts, this has been seen in a few animal trials, but much of the physiological effects of a longer rapid period have not been replicated in research studies.
- **Heart health:** Fasting over a short period increases blood pressure, sleeping heart rates, and other heart-related metrics.
- **Diabetes and obesity;** Intermittent Fasting has been shown to inhibit obesity in animals. In six small trials, obese adult humans shed weight by fasting intermittently.
- **Thinking and memory;** Intermittent Fasting improves working memory in livestock or verbal memory in adults, according to research.
- **Physical performance:** Fasting for 16 hours resulted in weight reduction while retaining muscle mass in young males. Mice that were fed on different days had greater running stamina.
- **Tissue health:** Intermittent Fasting in animals minimized tissue injury during treatment and increased outcomes.

1.5 Is Intermittent Fasting Safe?

A few people use Intermittent Fasting to lose weight, while others use it to treat serious illnesses, including irritable bowel syndrome, elevated cholesterol, as well as arthritis. Intermittent Fasting, on the other hand, isn't for all. Before attempting intermittent Fasting (or another diet), nutritionists recommend consulting with your general practitioner.

Any individuals must avoid experimenting with intermittent Fasting:
- Children and teenagers under the age of eighteen.
- Women who are expecting a child or who are breastfeeding.
- Diabetics and those with blood sugar issues.
- People who have had an eating problem in the past.

People who aren't in these ranges yet can successfully do intermittent Fasting can maintain the diet forever, according to experts. It may be a beneficial improvement in one's lifestyle. Consider that intermittent Fasting may have a variety of consequences depending on the person. If you have unusual distress, headaches, nausea, or other signs after beginning intermittent Fasting, see your doctor.

FASTING HASN'T BEEN LINKED TO ANY HEALTH ISSUES.

Although evidence shows that Fasting may help with a variety of illnesses, like multiple sclerosis and asthma, physicians recommend that if you're physically qualified to fast comfortably (which excludes those with more severe health issues), so there is no research to indicate why you shouldn't. We don't have proof that Fasting is unhealthy if you're not on pharmaceutical drugs, are relatively well, and choose to do so regularly because you believe it benefits your health. According to research on the topic, a study found that there were no specific risks associated with intermittent fasting diets. Still, the writers of that study point out that long-term evidence on the sustainability of intermittent Fasting has yet to be gathered because it's unclear if those diets impact people in the long run.

Let's go into the basics before we get into the benefits of Fasting. Anyone thinking about undertaking a fasting diet must consult their doctor first, according to experts. Fasting regimes may be dangerous whether you have a history of eating disorders, asthma, low blood pressure (hypotension), and anemia; you're pregnant or nursing; you're on any prescribed drugs, or you have some medical conditions. Be sure the doctor is mindful of all medications you're taking, including over-the-counter medications and nutritional supplements, before you speak with them. On an empty stomach, a seemingly harmless drug like Tylenol (acetaminophen) may be dangerous. Finally, before you begin, read the fine print. On days that you're heavily limiting calories, you might need to change the exercise level and workload because you'll feel tired and grumpy, and you'll be more likely to faint. Fasting can be done on weekends and vacations rather than throughout the week, experts advise.

Not everybody can (or must) participate in IF. Pregnant women or those planning to become pregnant (longer fasting cycles can throw off the menstrual cycle), diabetics (blood sugar may drop too low in the absence of hunger), and those on various medications (food, or lack thereof, can impair absorption and dosage) are among others that shouldn't. Often, if you have an experience of an eating disorder, adding times where you're "not permitted" to eat might set you up for a serious relapse. It's important to be aware that IF has any side effects. During fasting times, you can be irritable; "hanger" is real; low blood sugar may screw with your mood. When you do feed, you would want to eat a balanced diet.

One theory is that if you fasted for a couple of days, it would be impossible to make up a calorie deficiency, but in our world, with accessibility to calorie-dense foods, you could easily manage it. Concentrate on nutrient-dense foods such as apples, tomatoes, healthy fats, legumes, or whole grains (though some experts also pair IF with low-carb or keto styles of eating). Expect to experience low capacity, bloating, and cravings within the first few weeks as the body changes.

If you are the following groups of individuals, you can stop them:

- **People with diabetes**
  According to a study released, while IF can increase insulin sensitivity and thus be helpful for people with type 2 diabetes, it may also be dangerous for people taking diabetes drugs that cause hypoglycemia (low blood sugar), like insulin. As a result, people with type 1 diabetes who depend on insulin can avoid IF.

- **Underweight people**
  According to a study released, those with a BMI of less than 18.5 are not recommended to try weight reduction diets that include IF.

- **People with a current or a history of eating disorders**
  If you eat infrequently, you might develop an unhealthy diet. Any people could be inclined to use the conclusion of their fast as an opportunity to gorge on fatty snacks, according to a recent report.

- **People with other chronic diseases**
  Fasting's impact on certain chronic conditions, including diabetes, remains unknown, although negative side effects, including dizziness and nausea, might be more noticeable in certain patients. When you have medical problems that may be exacerbated by not feeding properly, you must be cautious.

- **Elderly people**
  Fasting has been linked to an increased incidence of stroke, cardiovascular disease, or arrhythmia in the elderly.

WOMEN WHO ARE PREGNANT OR BREASTFEEDING

Breastfeeding isn't the safest time to hurry or cut calories, according to a survey, so women require an additional 300 to 500 calories each day to maintain levels of energy and milk output. People who must take medicine with food can still feed at daily hours to avoid missing a dose. Before beginning a fast, everybody can consult with a specialist, whether they have either of the conditions mentioned above. Fasting may pose a danger to pregnant women, so they should seek medical advice before embarking on any program. Intermittent Fasting has few negative consequences for a fit, well-nourished human. As the body responds to Fasting, an individual can feel somewhat mentally and physically sluggish at first. Most citizens return to regular functioning after the change. People with medical problems, on the other hand, can contact their doctor before starting any fasting program.

The following people are especially vulnerable to Fasting and could need medical supervision:

- Those who are struggling to start a family
- Individuals who have trouble controlling their blood sugar levels
- Those suffering from a serious disorder such as heart failure or type 2 diabetes
- Women who are struggling to get pregnant

- Women who are expecting a child or who are breastfeeding
- Underweight individuals
- People who have struggled with an eating condition
- All who have a low blood pressure
- Individuals who take prescribed drugs
- Women who have had a diagnosis of amenorrhea
- Seniors
- Children

Although fasting may be beneficial to certain people, whether you have some medical problems or are pregnant, breastfeeding, or attempting to conceive, you should see your doctor first. Fasting is not advised by those who previously struggled with an eating condition. Fasting is the ritual of going without food or drink for a prolonged amount of time. It could improve your well-being depending on how it's handled. Fasting should be done for food, political, or religious reasons. Intermittent Fasting is a common practice that involves cycling through cycles of feeding and fasting. It's safest to keep fasting times brief, stop strenuous activity, and remain hydrated while fasting. When you're not fasting, eating enough protein, and maintaining a healthy diet will help you improve your overall health and ensure a good early.

Chapter 2.
How Intermittent Fasting Works

Forget about measuring calories or avoiding carbs; the new food craze allows you to consume whatever you want, but it concentrates on when you consume. Intermittent Fasting is a form of eating that has climbed the ranks of mainstream diets in recent years, being one of the most searched diets on Google, with hundreds of thousands of requests every month on average. What is the source of its ubiquity? For certain individuals, it seems to be a lot smoother. Traditional lifestyle improvements also depend on calorie counting, point tracking, or rules, which may seem like a lot of work and commitment for certain people, particularly those with busy lives or who are pulled in a lot of directions. But it's a lot simpler for them to maintain in this situation when what they must do is miss a meal.

2.1 How Does Intermittent Fasting Work?

Intermittent Fasting may be done in a variety of forms. However, most of them revolve around eating and fasting at regular intervals. You should, for example, just eat for eight hours a day and fast the rest of the time. Alternatively, you might opt to consume just one meal a day for two days a week. Intermittent Fasting can be done in a variety of ways. According to experts, the body's sugar reserves are depleted after many hours without calories, and the body begins to burn fat. Metabolic switching is how experts respond to it. Intermittent Fasting is in comparison to the typical diet routine among most Americans, who feed continuously throughout the day. If you consume three meals a day and snacks and don't work out, you're eating calories rather than burning fat stores.

Intermittent Fasting works by lengthening the interval between meals before the body has consumed enough of the calories and can begin losing fat. Fasting, often referred to as prolonged Fasting, focuses on what you prepare rather than what you consume. It isn't about calorie reduction for days on end; instead, it's about feeding for a set number of hours per day or some days a week and only refraining or reducing food intake over a set amount of time. For example, the Fast Diet, often recognized as the 5:2 diet, recommends consuming anything you like for five days of the week (without much attention to calorie consumption) and limiting calorie consumption to 500 calories for females and 600 calories for males for the remaining two days of the week (roughly one-quarter of the diet's "law of thumb" calorie intake for non-fasting days). Your body responds as you limit your calorie intake. Your digestive system converts carbohydrates into glucose, the body's primary source of energy, while you feed. Glucose is ingested into the bloodstream and then transported to the cells of the body to supply fuel.

When you don't consume food, the following effects may occur:

- If the levels of sugar in your blood decrease, your body can begin to depend on glycogen, or stored glucose, for energy.
- When the glycogen in your body is depleted, the body starts to burn muscle and fat to provide glucose for your cells.
- Your body enters a ketosis state after a few days without feeding (which doctors don't recommend), which means it burns fat as the primary source of fuel while sparing muscle.
- When you're in ketosis, you'll lose weight by burning body fat. Ketosis causes the blood to become more acidic, which may lead to poor breath, nausea, and other painful symptoms. Fasting for longer periods will damage the kidneys and liver.

Although so-called fasting diets have grown in popularity, Fasting is not a recent concept. Fasting has traditionally been a feature of religious rituals, and the ability to go without eating over long periods is an essential part of human development. Human bodies are prepared to withstand times of not feeding, thanks to our past as hunter-gatherers. Since our ancestors who made it through those hard times are the ones who lived, our DNA may be programmed to profit from Fasting.

2.2 Burning Questions About Intermittent Fasting

Forget about measuring calories or avoiding carbs; the new food craze allows you to consume whatever you want, but it concentrates on when you consume. Intermittent Fasting is a form of eating that has climbed the ranks of mainstream diets in recent years, being one of the most searched diets on Google, with hundreds of thousands of requests every month on average. What is the source of its ubiquity? For certain individuals, it seems to be a lot smoother. Traditional lifestyle improvements also depend on calorie counting, point tracking, or rules, which may seem like a lot of work and commitment for certain people, particularly those with busy lives or who are pulled in a lot of directions. But it's a lot simpler for them to maintain in this situation when what they must do is miss a meal. Here, we'll go through the fundamentals of IF and address all your burning questions.

What Is the History of Intermittent Fasting?

Fasting has been around since the beginning of time and is often associated with faith. However, the current iteration of IF emerged in the last eight years or so. The impressive advantages of Intermittent Fasting have been shown by extensive studies over the last five years, which is behind this sudden demand.

HOW DOES INTERMITTENT FASTING WORK?

There are a few different variations of IF (described below), but they all adopt the same general principle of classifying a specific time of the week for eating as well as a specific time of the week for restricting meals and drinks (or severely limited).

2.3 CAN INTERMITTENT FASTING HELP YOU LOSE WEIGHT?

The short response is most likely. IF has received a lot of attention as a weight-loss aid, and many experts advocate it in their weight-loss and weight-management practices. According to Harvard Health, it's related to weight loss because not eating in between meals causes the body to depend on fat contained in cells for energy. Insulin levels fall when the body loses fat in this step. Although, according to experts, all it boils down to is calorie restriction. As opposed to eating every day, people prefer to ingest fewer calories in a shorter period, which contributes to weight loss. In a survey affecting 23 obese people, it was discovered that those who followed the 16:8 solution to IF consumed around 300 fewer calories per day. Nighttime feeding has been found to lead to metabolic syndrome and obesity, so versions of IF that limit eating after a specific time, like 7 p.m., can help prevent it. However, some experts argue that the amount of weight reduction achieved by IF is comparable to that achieved by other calorie-restrictive diets. After one year, a report showed that a diet that reduced calories by 20% resulted in comparable weight loss to the 5:2 variant of IF. Still, if you find it simpler to adhere to than other diets, IF could be a smart choice.

2.4 WHAT IF CAN AND CAN'T DO FOR YOUR HEALTH

Further study is needed, although several findings show that fasting or restricting the intake of food for an amount of time may provide a lot of health benefits. Search "fasting for fitness," and you'll get over 6.3 million results, varying from physicians who prescribe this for a variety of ailments to spas that offer detoxifying food-free holidays to internet sources that claim that Fasting helps them feel more emotionally calm and physically healthy, and, gradually, to exercise pros touting programs that include fasting as a tool for losing weight. Is medical science, though, able to back up these assertions? Organs like the liver, kidneys, and spleen function tirelessly every day to eliminate and neutralize contaminants from the body to keep our cells safe. Fasting removes extra chemicals from the body, which can have biochemical benefits." The main term here is "potential." While a growing body of evidence indicates intermittent Fasting has health benefits, most of the evidence is still inconclusive, and there are several unknowns regarding how a fasting diet or intermittent fasting diet could affect our bodies in the long run.

How is IF different from Starvation?

Fasting (or a substantial decrease in calorie intake) and feeding at set hours are alternated in the intermittent fasting (IF) diet. It differs from most diets in that regard. It does not include the use of ingredients. It's also not about deprivation with IF. Rather, it entails taking the food at specific times and fasting the remainder of the day and night.

2.5 MAINTAINING INTERMITTENT FASTING

Intermittent Fasting can be made possible with yoga and moderate workouts. Maintaining an intermittent fasting regimen may be difficult.

The following suggestions will help people keep on board and get the most out of intermittent Fasting:

- **Keep yourself hydrated.** Throughout the day, consume plenty of water and calorie-free beverages like herbal teas.
- **Keeping diet from being an obsession**. On fasting days, plan lots of distractions to keep you from worrying about food, such as keeping up on paperwork or heading to the movies.
- **Resting and unwinding on fasting days,** avoid strenuous exercises, while light exercise such as yoga can be helpful.
- **Each calorie is counted**. Choose nutrient-dense meals that are high in protein, fiber, and healthy fats if the preferred schedule requires any calories during fasting times. Corn, lentils, eggs, chicken, almonds, and avocado are only a few examples.
- **Consuming goods that are more in volume**. Popcorn, fresh veggies, and fruits with strong water content, such as grapes and melon, are also good choices for filling low-calorie foods.
- **Increasing flavor without adding calories**. Garlic, vegetables, sauces, or vinegar may be used liberally to season meals. These foods are very low in calories but high in taste, which can help to alleviate hunger pangs.
- **After the fasting time, use nutrient-dense foods**. Consuming diets rich in fiber, vitamins, minerals, and other nutrients helps to maintain blood sugar levels to avoid nutritional shortages. A well-balanced diet will help you lose weight and improve your general health.

Intermittent Fasting may be done in a variety of forms, though no plan can succeed for everybody. Individuals can have the greatest outcomes if they experiment with different models to see which best suits their lifestyle and desires. Fasting over long periods while the body is unprepared, regardless of the form of intermittent Fasting, may be troublesome. These diets might not be enough for all. These approaches can worsen a person's unhealthy relationship with food if they are susceptible to disordered eating. Before undertaking some sort of Fasting, people with health problems, such as diabetes, can see a doctor. On non-fasting days, it's important to consume a healthy, nutritious diet for the best outcomes. An individual should obtain clinical assistance if appropriate to personalize an intermittent fasting schedule and prevent pitfalls.

HOW TO BEGIN INTERMITTENT FASTING?

Here's how it works:

- It's important to note that Intermittent Fasting is not a diet. It is a method of eating that is timed. Intermittent Fasting, unlike a dietary schedule that limits where calories come from, does not prescribe which foods an individual can consume or avoid. While intermittent Fasting has certain health benefits, like weight loss, it is not for everybody. Intermittent Fasting entails cycling between feeding and fasting times.
- People can find it daunting at first to eat just for a brief period per day or to switch between eating and not eating days. This will offer you advice about how to get started fasting, such as setting personal targets, preparing menus, and determining calorie requirements.
- Intermittent Fasting is a common strategy for achieving the following goals:
- simplify their life
- lose weight
- improve their overall health and well-being, such as minimizing the effects of aging

Fasting is generally suitable for most fit, well-nourished citizens, although it might not be sufficient for those with medical conditions. The following tips are intended to assist those who are ready to begin fasting in making it as simple and successful as practicable.

PICK THE METHOD

Before attempting another fasting process, an individual can usually stay with one for at least a month. When it comes to fasting for health benefits, there are four options to consider. An individual should choose the plan that best fits their needs and that they believe they will be able to adhere to.

There are some of them:

- Eat Stop Eat
- Warrior Diet
- Lean gains
- Alternate Day Fasting

Before attempting a new fasting technique, an individual can usually stay with one for a month or longer to see how it works for them. Before starting any fasting process, someone with a medical condition can consult their doctor. When choosing a method, keep in mind that you don't have to consume a particular quantity or kind of food or skip certain foods entirely. An individual is free to consume whatever they want. During the feeding times, though, it is a smart idea to consume a balanced, high-fiber, vegetable-rich diet to achieve wellness and weight loss targets. On eating days, bingeing on unhealthy foods will sabotage your well-being. On the swift days, it's often important to consume plenty of water or other low-calorie drinks.

IDENTIFY PERSONAL GOALS

An individual who begins intermittent Fasting usually has a specific target in mind. That may be for weight loss, better physical health, or better metabolic function. A person's overall objective can aid them in determining the best fasting approach and calculating how many calories and nutrients they need.

2.6 EXERCISING WHILE INTERMITTENT FASTING

One hypothesis, according to Harvard Health, is that exercising when fasting will help burn fat. According to experts, the body needs sugar or any other source of energy to do well when exercising. Sugar ions, which are processed as glycogen in the liver, provide energy in most cases. Once you start running, certain supplies are more likely to be depleted, and the body would have no alternative but to move through a more anaerobic collapse to provide you with the resources you need.

Your body is pushed to burn off another energy source: fat instead of carbohydrates that aren't visible. However, you can lack the stamina to exercise as vigorously as you usually will. It is much simpler to achieve peak results or simply feel healthy when exercising if you diet. Intermittent Fasting does not impair the desire to exercise in healthier people, even during the time that the body adjusts to the new eating plan. An individual should not experience any negative effects from fasting on their exercise routine after the transition time.

Many are concerned about muscle loss when fasting can ingest adequate protein during feeding cycles and engage in daily resistance training. Fasting is less likely to cause muscle loss if protein consumption is maintained. Fasting is a normal part of life for humans. Most individuals have unwittingly fasted in their lives by enjoying a late dinner and missing food the following day. Some people can benefit from more formal approaches. However, while such items are not required to be excluded from a person's diet, they can also strive to consume a well-balanced diet rich in protein, fiber, and vegetables. Also, don't forget to drink lots of water. Finally, although the normal individual is unlikely to have any or just minor adverse effects, individuals with certain medical problems or who are taking any prescriptions should consult a doctor before embarking on a fasting regimen.

2.7 What's the Best Way to Manage Hunger While Fasting?

When the body responds to IF, you will most definitely feel hunger, but Gottfried claims that this will pass. It gets better, based on my own knowledge and that of my patients. IF does not raise total appetite, according to research. According to experts, the 16:8 diet (or a combination of it) seems to be the simplest for most people to incorporate into their daily lives without getting hungry.

What Side Effects Can You Expect on an Intermittent Fasting Diet?

Transitioning to this form of eating is difficult for many individuals. According to a 2019 study, Intermittent Fasting may trigger migraines, dizziness, nausea, and insomnia. It may even make people feel hungry and tired during the day, restricting their movement. According to the same report, calorie restriction could cause some women to quit menstruating. It's time to see a specialist if you skip three times in a row.

Best Way to Break a Fast and Begin Eating Again

Don't use the conclusion of the fast as an opportunity to binge on fatty foods; this could jeopardize the diet's chances of performance. Whether it's a regular overnight fast or a time-restricted diet, the fundamentals of healthy food and breaking a fast remain the same. Break the fast with a nutritious, balanced meal that includes lean proteins, complex carbohydrates, and healthy fats.

Protein should be given special consideration, particularly if you have diabetes. We often suggest eating a type of protein with every meal, particularly when breaking a fast, for people with diabetes to maintain regular sugar levels and prevent worsening insulin resistance. Protein does not break down into glucose as quickly as carbohydrates, but it affects blood sugar levels more slowly and gradually. Breaking the fast with a good supply of carbohydrates, according to experts, will help regenerate reduced glycogen amounts.

They suggest a Mediterranean-style meal that contains 40% carbs, 30% protein, and 30% fat. Experts still believe that the order in which you split your fast will make a difference. People who consume their calories later in the day, even though they are the same number of calories, weigh more than those who eat them early in the day, according to reports. According to a report, sleep-deprived people with late bedtimes are more likely to add weight since the foods they consume at night are richer in fat than those they eat throughout the day. When assessing you're eating window, keep this in mind.

How to break your fast?

Are you thinking of incorporating intermittent Fasting into your low-carb, keto diet to boost your weight reduction and metabolic improvements? Then you may be considering how to sever your fasts in the most effective way possible.

- *What do you think you should eat first?*
- *What produces the highest outcomes?*
- *What can you be on the lookout for?*

Whether you're new to Fasting or have already struggled to break a fast, this guide will help you prepare and follow the right ways to resume eating after a fast or longer fast.

Fasting: New twist on an old tradition

Historically, the term "breakfast" referred to the very first food of the day, regardless of where it happened. It wasn't until the 15th century that the term came to mean the first thing you eat after waking up. With the rise of extended Fasting, the sense of the expression "breakfast" is returning to its origins. Breakfast is the meal eaten as you want to break your fast, whether it's at 6:00 a.m. or 6:00 p.m. Fasting has been practiced for centuries, particularly for religious reasons. And, for the most part, how to crack the fast was not given any thought in human history. However, in an era with bad nutritional recommendations, where we are advised to snack every day, and where hyper-palatable heavily packaged food abounds, resuming eating in a manner that achieves the best physical ease and most successful outcomes with the long-term well-being and weight loss objectives can require a little more preparation.

2.8 The Difference Between Short and Long Fasts

We go into a short-term fast every night as we finish eating and go to bed before our first meal the next day. You will comfortably go on a 12 to 16-hour fast depending on when you consumed dinner and when you eat the first meal after waking up, with no physiologic changes to digestive functions. Although there is no specific agreement or agreed concept about what constitutes a short or long-term fast, the Diet Doctor describes time-restricted eating as anything less than 24 hours, short-term fasts as 24 to 36 hours, and long-term fasts as more than 36 hours. When it comes to time-restricted feeding and short-term fasts, there are no special steps to take when it comes to breaking the fast. It's important to note that bingeing on heavily refined, sugary, or high-carb foods can negate the benefits of the fast. Prepare a nutritious, low-carb, high-fat recipe.

ENDING A LONGER FAST: A QUIET GUT REVS UP AGAIN.

Fasting over longer periods is different. Resuming feeding after a longer fast necessitates further forethought and consideration. When we begin to integrate fasting into our daily lives, our bodies take some time to adapt to the new schedule, particularly if we have been eating continuously. As pathological eaters, our bodies expend metabolic energy to produce digestive enzymes to absorb the food we eat. When we first begin fasting, this improves. There is no requirement for our production of digestive enzymes.

POTENTIAL SIDE EFFECTS OF BREAKING A LONG-TERM FAST

If you've been fasting for a long time and your body's natural output of gastric juice has slowed, you may feel gastrointestinal discomfort when you eat again.

This is usually expressed as:

- Diarrhea or loose stools
- Passing of undigested foods
- Gas pains
- Bloating
- In very rare cases, nausea, and vomiting

Food will stay in your stomach for even longer when your body doesn't have the digestive enzymes and juices it needs to break down right away. It can take many hours or even days for your body to begin producing the enzymes used to break it down. You can start to feel abdominal pains during this time. Aside from cutting the length of the hard, the only approach to reduce side effects is to prepare the best things to consume when you split it.

Chapter 3.
INTERMITTENT FASTING FOR ELDERLY WOMEN

Intermittent Fasting is one of the most common diets right now. Fans say it will help with weight loss, lose fat, lower blood pressure, and reduce the risk of diabetes. With all these alleged advantages, people, especially women, could wonder whether they should try Intermittent Fasting. People also traditionally fasted for religious purposes. However, in modern years, more have hopped on an intermittent fasting bandwagon because of the potential health benefits. While there is some evidence to support these claims, Intermittent Fasting has been seen to have detrimental effects on women's hormones, fertility, as well as bone health. The diet's restricting aspect can often lead to disordered feeding. Here, we look at the research regarding intermittent Fasting, what it is, what it can do for you, what the advantages are, what the risks are, and how to get involved. In past years, Intermittent Fasting has grown in popularity. Intermittent eating, unlike other diets, relies on what to feed by adding daily short-term fasts into the schedule. This eating style can assist you in consuming fewer calories, losing weight, and reducing your risk of diabetes and risk of heart disease. Intermittent Fasting, on the other hand, could not be as effective for women as it is for men, according to a variety of reports. As a result, women will need to take a different path. While intermittent Fasting has several advantages, it can be harmful to women. We go through the advantages and disadvantages of intermittent Fasting for females, as well as how to get started.

3.1 INTERMITTENT FASTING FOR WOMEN

Intermittent Fasting (IF) is an eating practice that alternates between times of Fasting and periods of regular eating. Fasting on alternating days, occasional 16-hour fasts, and fasting for 24 hours two days a week are the most popular practices. Both intermittent fasting regimens would be referred to as intermittent Fasting in this report. Intermittent Fasting, unlike other diets, does not require calorie or macronutrient monitoring. There are no dietary or dietary restrictions, making it more like behavior than a meal. Intermittent Fasting is a popular method to lose weight since it is an easy, fast, and inexpensive way to eat less or lose body fat. Its growth also aids in the prevention of diabetes and heart disease, the maintenance of muscle strength, and the improvement of psychological well-being. Furthermore, since there are fewer meals to schedule, prepare, and serve, this eating style will help you save time in the kitchen. Intermittent Fasting is a form of eating that involves periodic, short-term Fasting. It's a common way of living that can help with disease prevention, weight loss, body composition, and overall well-being. Time-restricted IF entails only feeding during a specific time frame, like the 16:8, in which you feed for 8 hours (normally 12–08 p.m.) but then fast during the remaining 16 hours. Few people adapt by fasting for 12 hours and only eating throughout a 12-hour timeframe. The 5:2 diet, also known as adapted Fasting, entails limiting calories to 20-25 percent of daily energy requirements on two non - consecutive days a week (as little as 500 calories a day), with no calorie or pacing limits on the remaining five days. Fasting days (when you don't eat at all) are alternated with non-fasting days in a full alternate-day fast (eating anything you like).

3.2 INTERMITTENT FASTING MAY AFFECT MEN AND WOMEN DIFFERENTLY

Intermittent Fasting might not be as effective for several women as it is for men, according to some facts. In one research, women's blood sugar regulation deteriorated after three weeks of intermittent Fasting, while men's blood sugar control improved. There have also been several observational reports about women's menstrual cycles changing since they began Intermittent Fasting. Since female bodies are particularly vulnerable to calorie restriction, such changes arise. A small portion of the brain called the hypothalamus is impaired when calorie consumption is limited, such as when fasting for too long or too often. Gonadotropin-releasing hormone (GnRH) is a hormone that aids in the activation of two reproductive hormones: luteinizing hormone (LH) and follicle-stimulating hormone (FSH) (FSH). When these hormones are unable to interact with the ovaries, irregular cycles, miscarriage, poor bone strength, and other health problems may occur. While no equivalent human trials exist, 3 to 6 months of alternate-day Fasting in female rats resulted in a decrease in ovary size and erratic menstrual cycles. Women should take a changed solution to intermittent Fasting, like shorter fasting times and fewer fasting days, because of these factors. Women cannot benefit as much from intermittent Fasting as men do. Women can adopt a gentle approach to Fasting, with shorter fasts and fewer fasting days, to avoid the negative consequences.

3.3 IF FOR WOMEN AFTER 50

When it comes to losing weight, women over 50 will have a difficult time. This can be caused by a variety of factors. The most common cause is a slowed metabolism. Your metabolism will be quicker if you have more lean muscle. However, when we age, we reduce lean muscle mass and become less healthy than we once were.

What's the result?

Obstinate body fat that refuses to go away. Intermittent Fasting has grown in popularity in recent years because of its many health benefits and the fact that it does not limit your food options. Fasting has been shown to increase appetite, and mental well-being and potentially deter certain cancers, according to research. It may also protect women over 50 from some muscle, nerve, or joint disorders. Intermittent Fasting (IF) is essentially restricting the diet to a set period. There are several different types of IF to pick from. Choose the kind that better suits your lifestyle, and then discuss it with your practitioner.

DAILY METHOD

This is the most often used IF form. A 16/8 or 18/6 law is commonly used in the regular system. This entails consuming normal, nutritious meals for six to eight hours per day and then fasting for the other 16 to 18 hours. This has been discovered to be the most long-term form. To get started, experiment with different timing options. A 12/12 diet involves feeding for 12 hours and then fasting for 12 hours. When you're ready, you should move on to a more rigid timetable.

5:2 METHOD

This method entails consuming regular, nutritious meals five days a week and restricting oneself to 500 to 600 calories two days a week. It's uncertain if eating all the ones' calories in one sitting or spreading them out over the day is better, so do what is best for you.

ALTERNATE DAY METHOD

You could regularly eat any other day if you chose this form. On fasting days, you'll consume just 25% of the normal calorie requirements. For instance, if you normally consume 1,800 calories a day, you will consume just 450 calories on fasting days.

24-HOUR METHOD

Fasting for a complete 24 hours before eating again is needed for this process. Fasting from bed to breakfast or lunch to dinner is normally performed once or twice a week by those who use this form. If you use this form, proceed with caution. It may trigger extreme irritability, nausea, and headaches, and this approach might or may not be best for you. It can be odd that merely changing your eating schedule will help you lose weight. About this, our bodies adapt to fasting positively. When your body goes into fasting mode, your fat reserves are called upon to be used as food, allowing you to consume fat for energy. Of course, just because you aren't fasting doesn't suggest you should eat whatever you want. To get the best outcomes, eat balanced whole grains, unrefined carbs, and lean proteins. During fasting times, you should also consume calorie-free beverages like black coffee, tea, or water. You might also note that you are feeding more slowly and for greater enjoyment. The benefits of IF go beyond weight reduction. Fasting has been performed in several countries since ancient times, although it is now done daily in others. Health advantages are a positive side effect of IF, and most of them are beneficial to women's health.

WHO SHOULDN'T TRY INTERMITTENT FASTING?

Irregular fasting isn't suitable for anyone. Before beginning every new diet, including one that is beneficial, you should still consult a doctor.

If you belong to one of the following parties, you can stop it:

- Those may have diabetes and other insulin level issues.
- Minors under the age of eighteen.
- People who have had an eating problem in the past.
- Mothers who are pregnant or breastfeeding.

3.4 HEALTH BENEFITS OF INTERMITTENT FASTING FOR WOMEN

Intermittent fasting will help you lose weight while still lowering the chance of contracting a variety of diseases.

HEART HEALTH

The main cause of death in the world is heart failure. High blood pressure, higher LDL cholesterol, and high triglyceride levels are three of the most common risks for cardiac failure. Intermittent fasting reduced blood pressure by 6 percent in only eight weeks in a sample of sixteen obese men and women. Intermittent fasting also reduced LDL cholesterol by 25 percent or triglycerides by 32%, according to the same report. The evidence for a correlation between intermittent fasting and lower LDL cholesterol and triglycerides, on the other hand, is mixed. Four weeks of intermittent fasting over the Islamic holiday of Ramadan did not result in a decrease in LDL cholesterol or triglycerides, according to a survey of 40 normal-weight individuals. Until researchers completely comprehend the impact of intermittent fasting on cardiac health, higher-quality experiments with more rigorous methods are needed.

DIABETES

Intermittent fasting will also help you treat your diabetes and lower your chances of contracting it. Intermittent fasting, including prolonged calorie restriction, tends to reduce some diabetes risk factors. It mostly accomplishes this by lowering insulin levels and decreasing insulin tolerance. Six months of intermittent fasting cut insulin levels by 29% and insulin tolerance by 19% in a randomized controlled trial of more than 100 overweight or obese women. The amounts of blood sugar stayed unchanged. Furthermore, intermittent fasting for 8–12 weeks has been found to decrease insulin levels by 20–31 percent and blood glucose levels by 3–6 percent in people with pre-diabetes, a disease wherein blood sugar levels are high but not severe enough to make a diagnosis. In terms of blood sugar, though, intermittent fasting might not be as effective for females as it is for males. A small study showed that women's blood sugar balance deteriorated throughout 22 days of alternative fasting, although men's blood sugar levels were unaffected. Considering this risk factor, the decrease in insulin and insulin tolerance will possibly reduce the incidence of diabetes, particularly in pre-diabetic individuals.

WEIGHT LOSS

When performed correctly, intermittent fasting can be an easy and efficient way to reduce weight since short-term fasts can let you eat fewer calories and lose weight. Several reports have found that intermittent fasting is just as successful as conventional calorie-restricted diets for weight loss in the short term. Intermittent fasting resulted in an overall weight reduction of 15 lbs. (6.8 kg) over 3–12 months, according to a 2018 study of research in overweight adults. Over 3–24 weeks, intermittent fasting decreased body weight by 3–8% in overweight or obese individuals, according to another study. Participants' waist circumference decreased by 3–7% during the same period, according to the report. It's worth noting that the long-term consequences of intermittent fasting on female weight loss are also unknown. Intermittent starvation seems to help with weight reduction in the short term. The amount you lose, though, can most definitely be determined by how many calories you eat during non-fasting hours and how long you stick to the lifestyle.

IT MAY HELP YOU EAT LESS

Transitioning to intermittent fasting may help you eat less naturally. When young men's food consumption was limited to a four-hour duration, they consumed 650 fewer calories per day, according to one report. Another research looked at the impact of a lengthy, 36-hour fast on the eating patterns of 24 active men and women. Despite eating more calories on the post-fast day, participants' overall calorie balance fell by 1,900 calories, a substantial decrease.

3.5 FOOD CHOICES FOR ENDING LONGER FASTS

You should stop consuming things that are hard on the system until the body knows that you aren't stressed and are just eating less often. Some individuals are certain that such foods irritate their stomachs more than others. If you have an issue with those ingredients, you can stop them when you first start eating again.

In general, we've discovered that these foods (and drinks) are the most difficult for people to eat while they're breaking their fast, while some people handle them fine:

- Nut butter and nuts
- Seed butter and seeds
- Vegetables cruciferous, raw
- Eggs
- Dairy products
- Alcohol
- Few may experience trouble digesting red meat or certain types of red meat on special occasions.

You should be able to eat the food mentioned here without trouble within six hours of breaking your fast.

THE RECOMMENDED PROTOCOL FOR BREAKING A FAST

The following procedure, which we discovered in our Intensive Dietary Management Program, fits well for those who feel anxiety when breaking their fasts:

- Make sure you're well-hydrated before you begin.
- Begin your meal with a cup of chopped parsley with tomatoes and cucumber salad. When desired, tbsp of extra virgin olive oil may be added.
- Keep your protein sources to poultry or fish to be healthy. They can be fried in fat, and the skin of the chicken can be eaten. Try to keep the protein consumption to no more than the scale and thickness of your palm.
- Complete the remainder of the plate with non-starchy, above-ground veggies fried in healthy fats such as avocado, cocoa butter, butter, or clarified butter.
- If you're ever hungry, add avocado at the end of your meal.

If you still have trouble following this treatment, try a tablespoon of psyllium husk in a cup of water. Some people find it beneficial, although others believe it causes bloating. If it works, try the above treatment the next time you're fasting and about to restart feeding. However, apply a tablespoon of psyllium to the water at the beginning.

A WORD ABOUT ALCOHOL

When breaking a fast of more than 36 hours, it's critical to avoid alcohol, particularly binge drinking. Alcoholic ketoacidosis is characterized by a large level of ketones in the blood. However, unlike diabetic ketoacidosis, blood glucose levels are normally dangerously normal. Vomiting and stomach discomfort are the most common conditions. It is more frequent in individuals who have alcohol addictions or a heavy dependency on alcohol and who go days without eating before drinking heavily. It has, however, been identified in people of all ages who have consumed a large amount of alcohol with little too little food.

3.6 EFFECTIVENESS OF INTERMITTENT FASTING

Fasting has many physiological impacts on a person's body. Here are some of the effects:

- Insulin levels are reduced, making it simpler for the body to burn accumulated fat.
- Blood sugar, blood pressure, and inflammatory levels are also reduced.
- Changing the expression of specific genes, aids in disease prevention and survival.
- Human growth hormone, or HGH, is a hormone that aids in the use of body fat and the growth of muscle.
- Autophagy is a term used by physicians to describe a regeneration mechanism in which the body digests or recycles old or weakened cell components.

Fasting may be traced back to early people, who would sometimes go hours or days without eating due to a lack of calories. The human body adapted to this eating style by having longer gaps between meals. This compulsory Fasting is recreated by Intermittent Fasting. Intermittent Fasting for nutritional reasons may be very useful for weight reduction. Most people attempt Intermittent Fasting to lose weight, according to one survey. Other literature supports the argument that Fasting will aid weight loss. According to a study of research, several individuals who fast have a greater loss in visceral body fat and a comparable to a marginally lower decrease of body weight than others who practice more conventional calorie-reduction diets. Fasting has also been shown to be useful in the control of metabolic syndrome and diabetes, as well as extending lifetime, protecting neuron activity, and showing potential in the treatment of digestive diseases, according to research.

OTHER HEALTH BENEFITS

Intermittent fasting can also have other health effects, according to a variety of animal and human reports.

- **Reduced inflammation:** Intermittent fasting has been shown in several trials to suppress essential markers of inflammation. Chronic inflammation can trigger weight gain and a slew of other health issues.
- **Improved psychological well-being:** In one report, eight weeks of intermittent fasting reduced stress and binge eating habits in obese adults, thus enhancing body appearance.
- **Increased longevity:** Intermittent fasting has been used to extend lifespan by 33–83 percent in rats and mice. The impact on human survival is still to be calculated.
- **Preserve muscle mass:** When opposed to prolonged calorie restriction, intermittent fasting tends to be more efficient at maintaining muscle mass. And when you're at rest, having more muscle mass makes you eat more calories. Before any findings may be made, the health effects of intermittent fasting for females must be investigated more thoroughly in well-designed human trials. Intermittent fasting can aid weight loss and lower the risk of heart disease or diabetes in women. However, more human research is required to back up these results.

MUSCULOSKELETAL HEALTH

Osteoporosis, hypertension, and lower back discomfort are also examples of this. Fasting has been found to increase thyroid hormone secretion. This can help avoid bone breaks by promoting bone health.

METABOLIC HEALTH

Around their 50s, certain people experience menopause. Changes in the body during menopause will lead to a rise in belly fat, insulin, or glucose levels. Fasting will help you lose weight and increase insulin sensitivity by lowering blood pressure, cholesterol, or belly fat. Fasting will also help you maintain a healthy metabolism when you get older.

MENTAL HEALTH

Fasting is beneficial to one's emotional well-being. It can help with anxiety, and depression, as well as the emotional ups and downs that come with menopause. Fasting has been shown to boost self-esteem and lower stress levels. IF has already been seen to have the following advantages:

- Better recall
- Better tissue wellbeing
- Better physical output
- Cardiovascular wellbeing

3.7 BEST TYPES OF INTERMITTENT FASTING FOR WOMEN

There is no such thing as a one-size-fits-all solution to dieting. This is true with extended fasting as well. Women can, on average, take a more casual approach to fast than men. Shorter fasting times, fewer fasting days, and/or eating a limited number of calories on fasting days are also possible options. Here are a few of the better intermittent fasting options for women:

- **Crescendo Method**

Fasting for 12 to 16 hours twice or three times a week. Fasting days must not be concurrent and should be spread out uniformly during the week, such as Monday, Wednesday, and Friday.

- **Eat-stop-eat (also called the 24-hour protocol)**

Once or twice a week, go on a complete 24-hour easy (maximum of 2 times a week for women). Proceed with 14–16 hour fasts and work your way up.

- **The 5:2 Diet (also called "The Fast Diet")**

Two days a week, limit calories to 25 percent of your usual Diet (about 500 calories) and eat regularly the other five days. Fasting days can be separated by one day.

- **Modified Alternate-Day Fasting**

On non-fasting days, I feed "normally," but on fasting days, I eat "normally." On a fasting day, you are required to eat 20–25 percent of your normal calorie intake (roughly 500 calories).

- **The 16/8 Method (also called the "Lean gains method")**

Fasting for 16 hours a day and consuming all your calories in eight hours. Women can begin with 14-hour fasts and work their way up to 16 hours. It is also necessary to eat well during the non-fasting hours, regardless of which option you choose. You do not enjoy the same weight reduction and health effects if you consume a lot of fatty, calorie-dense items during non-fasting times. At the end of the day, the right solution is something that you can handle and maintain overtime without causing any detrimental health effects. Intermittent fasting may be done in a variety of forms by women. The 5:2 Diet adapted to alternate-day fasting, and the crescendo approach are three of the most effective approaches.

How to Get Started?

It's simple to get started. You've probably done a few sporadic fasts before. Often people eat this way out of habit, avoiding breakfast and dinner. The most straightforward approach to get started is to use one of the intermittent fasting techniques mentioned above. You may not, though, must stick to a strict schedule. Another choice is to fast anytime it is convenient for you. For certain individuals, skipping meals because they aren't hungry or don't have time to prepare may be beneficial. It doesn't matter the kind of fast you want at the end of the day. Finding a tool that fits well for you and your behavior is the most critical thing. The simplest way to get started is to use one of the approaches mentioned above. If you feel some negative side effects, stop immediately. For instance, doctors advise against Whether people who don't get proper sleep, don't consume properly or regularly, have erratic or missing periods, have thyroid disorders, have a background of present or previous disordered eating, are stressed, or have blood sugar problems.

Experts normally recommend feeding consistently, which is a great way to relieve tension in the body and keep blood sugar in check. Long-term commitment to intermittent fasting has not been studied. Start slowly if your practitioner or dietitian has given you permission. Fasting for only 12 or 14 hours overnight has been found in several trials to have metabolic effects, but it's good to note that you don't have to fast for Sixteen to eighteen hours to reap the benefits. They advise starting with a time-restricted approach rather than the 5:2, which cuts calories two days a week and allows people to overeat the rest of the time. To begin, determine how many hours it takes you to go from the time you stop eating at night to the time you begin eating the next day. To begin, try increasing your fast by one hour, then two hours, and so on. There are no calorie limits in time-restricted IF. We suggest consuming three nutritious meals a day, spread equally across the eating window, including calcium, high-fiber carbs, and good fats. Many who have never been major breakfast eaters can find it easier to wait until 10 or 11 a.m. to eat, whilst some get up hungry. The most crucial thing is to pay attention to your body and feed while hungry. Intermittent fasting can be challenging for women who exercise often. It would be difficult to fast if it is the time of the month and you are ravenous. We understand what you're thinking: can coffee help you crack your fast? Yeah, theoretically, whether there's something in it.

There are no calories in black coffee. But think of your objectives: are you trying to lose weight? If that's the case, keep in mind that IF doesn't cause much further weight reduction than a calorie deficiency, then a little creamer in your coffee is usually perfect. Are you using so to keep your blood sugar in check? If that's the case, maybe a caramel latte isn't the perfect way to start the day. Fasting is a practice that can never be mistaken for a strict diet. There's a lot to think about for women before beginning intermittent fasting. Women with asthma, eating problems, or who are pregnant, or nursing should avoid IF. If you decide to try it, start slowly, and pay careful attention to your appetite and satiety. If you're always hungry over the day or week, it's probably easier to get back into a more normal eating routine. Keep an eye out for signs like nausea, mood fluctuations, appetite, low energy, lack of focus, and a missed menstrual period. Throughout the day, you should feel fueled, energized, and fulfilled, not groggy and starving.

3.8 Safety and Side Effects

Many women tend to be healthy by using modified forms of intermittent fasting. On the other hand, a variety of studies have shown that fasting days will trigger hunger, mood fluctuations, loss of focus, decreased stamina, headaches, and bad breath. Women's menstrual cycles have also been said to have ceased whilst on an intermittent fasting diet, according to several reports on the internet.

Before attempting intermittent fasting, contact the doctor if you have a medical problem. Medical advice is especially relevant for women who:

- Also had an eating problem in the past.
- Have diabetes or suffer from low blood pressure daily.
- They are underweight, malnutrition, and deficient in nutrients.
- Are you expecting a child, are you breastfeeding, or are you planning to conceive?
- Suffer from infertility or have a diagnosis of anemia (missed periods).

Finally, intermittent fasting seems to have a favorable protection profile. However, if you have any complications, such as a lack of your menstrual period, you can quit instantly. Hunger-reduced stamina, headaches, and poor breath are also possible side effects of intermittent fasting. Before beginning an intermittent fasting program, women who are pregnant, planning to conceive, or have a record of eating disorders must seek medical advice. Intermittent fasting is a dietary practice that entails short-term fasts daily. Regular 14–16-hour fasts, the 5:2 Diet, or adapted alternate-day fasting are the safest for women. Although intermittent fasting has been seen to benefit heart health, diabetes, and weight loss in some women, some research suggests it can have harmful effects on fertility and blood sugar levels in others. Updated versions of intermittent fasting, on the other hand, tend to be healthier for most women and could be a better choice than longer or tougher fasts. Intermittent fasting is something to think about whether you're a woman trying to reduce weight or boost your well-being.

Pros of Intermittent Fasting for Women

There is a lot of evidence to back up the medicinal effects of fasting. Improved cellular fitness, improved metabolic indicators, and weight reduction are also possible health advantages. Intermittent fasting causes weight loss in women, but it doesn't cause much further weight loss than a calorie deficiency overall, according to studies. The structure of IF, on the other hand, makes it possible for certain people to limit their food consumption. Intermittent fasting will also help you lose weight. Blood sugar (glucose) increases when we feed, and insulin is discharged to transport sugar to our body for energy. Excess glucose is quickly processed. If you go 10-16 hours without eating, your body can begin to use fat reserves for power. Cellular repair happens in a fasted condition, according to research, and has been attributed to enhanced survival, lower cancer risk, lower inflammation, and better metabolism. However, several of the experiments are conducted on livestock, and further research on women is needed. There's still new evidence that feeding in time with your circadian clock helps you avoid chronic diseases. In other terms, limiting overnight feeding to eating within a 6–10-hour window throughout the day when it's light outside.

Cons of Intermittent Fasting for Women

Regardless of the research's findings, it's necessary to keep the meaning in mind and always note that it's not suitable for everybody. Intermittent fasting can be avoided by females of reproductive age because their bodies are more vulnerable to stressors, including extended fasting or caloric restriction. Intermittent fasting is a cause of stress on the individual in and of itself, and when combined with our everyday lives that are already full of chronic psychological, physiological, or environmental stressors, IF may do more harm than good. Fasting raises cortisol levels and may trigger blood sugar imbalances, insulin tolerance, lean muscle weakness, exhaustion, and thyroid dysfunction overtime. Fasting may reduce thyroid-stimulating hormone in the short term, but chronically elevated cortisol may limit thyroid hormone conversion. Fasting can also contribute to under-eating and has been shown to hurt female hormones. Intermittent fasting may induce a lack of menstrual period and interact with fertility through restricting calories. Read more on how our hormones are affected by what we consume. Fasting may contribute to bingeing or a period of restricting and overeating through increasing appetite and fascination with food. This is especially harmful to people who have eating disorders and who have a past of food restriction or disordered eating. Hunger hormones are produced as the body goes without food for an extended amount of time, which increases appetite. Doctors say they often see females misusing IF by missing breakfast and feeding late into the evening, which may interrupt hormonal cycles and lead to hormone imbalance. They also say that women who practice IF are utterly missing their bodies' biological hunger signals, which are neither physically nor mentally healthy. Doctors say they often see females misusing IF by missing breakfast or feeding late into the night, which may interrupt hormonal cycles and lead to hormone imbalance. They also say that women who pursue IF are utterly missing their bodies' physiological hunger signals, which are neither physically nor mentally healthy.

Chapter 4.
TYPES AND METHODS OF DOING INTERMITTENT FASTING

Intermittent fasting advocates argue that it is simpler to stick to than conventional calorie-controlled diets. Intermittent fasting is a personal experience for each individual, and various styles will serve different people. We'll go into the science behind the most common forms of intermittent fasting and offer advice about how to stick to it. Intermittent fasting may be done in a variety of ways, though different individuals choose different forms. Continue reading to learn about seven different ways to quickly intermittently. On days when you are not fasting, you can consume about all you want. However, if you want to lose weight and receive the nutrition you need, you can consume nutritious meals and avoid sweets and refined foods. You can consume very little to no food on fasting days. Every Other Day Diet, for example, recommends eating no more than 500 calories on each fast day. Another method, known as the 5:2 Fast Diet, entails consuming five days per week and fasting the remaining two, with women receiving almost 500 calories and men receiving almost 600. That's around a quarter of what you consume on days when you don't find it easy. It's up to you whether you consume certain calories all at once or spread them out over a few micro-meals during the day.

4.1 POPULAR WAYS TO DO INTERMITTENT FASTING

Intermittent fasting has been a common health movement in recent years. It's said to help people lose weight, boost their metabolic fitness, and maybe even live longer. This eating trend may be approached in a variety of ways. Any strategy has the potential to be successful but determining which one works better for you is a personal decision. Intermittent fasting can be done in a variety of forms. Intermittent fasting can be done in a variety of forms. The number of fast days and calorie allowances differ between the systems. Intermittent fasting entails going without food for a period, either completely or partly, before eating normally again. According to several pieces of research, this type of eating will help you lose weight, improve your fitness, and live longer.

THE 16/8 METHOD
The 16/8 process entails fasting for 14–16 hours a day and limiting your feeding window to 8 to 10 hours. You may consume two, three, or even four meals during the feeding time. The Lean gains protocol is another name for this procedure. It's as simple as not consuming something after dinner and missing breakfast to follow this fasting process. If you have your final meal at 8:00 p.m.8:00 p.m. and don't eat again before lunchtime the next day, you'll have fasted for 16 hours. Women are usually advised to fast for just 14–15 hours since they tend to perform well with shorter fasts. This approach can be difficult to adjust to at first for individuals who get hungry in the morning and like to consume breakfast. Many breakfast-skippers, on the other hand, feed in this manner instinctively. During the fast, you can drink water, coffee, as well as other low-calorie drinks to make you feel less hungry. It's important to focus on consuming nutritious foods across your eating window. If you eat a lot of fast food or consume an unhealthy number of calories, this approach will not succeed.

4.2 12 HOURS A DAY–FAST

Intermittent fasting can fit different people in different ways. The Diet's rules are easy to follow. Every day, a person must select and adhere to a twelve-hour fasting cycle. According to some studies, fasting for ten–to sixteen hours allows the body to burn excess fat into energy by releasing ketone bodies into circulation. This will assist you with losing weight. This form of fasting technique can be a good option for beginners. This is because the fasting duration is comparatively short, most of the intermittent fasting happens while sleeping, and the individual will consume nearly the same number of calories per day. The most convenient approach to complete this kind of fast is to have sleeping time during the fasting period. Somebody could, for example, fast between the hours of 6 p.m. and 6 a.m. They'd have to end dinner at 6 p.m. and stay before 6 a.m. to have breakfast, but they'd be asleep for most of the period in between.

4.3 5:2

This Diet entails regularly eating five days a week and limiting your calorie consumption to 500–600 calories on the remaining two days. The Fast is another name for this diet. On fasting days, women should utilize 500 calories, and males should consume 600 calories. You can, for example, regularly eat every day except Mondays or Thursdays. You consume two minor meals of 250 calories each for females and 300 calories each for males for those two days. No trials are evaluating this diet specifically, as opponents rightly point out, but there are loads of studies about the advantages of intermittent fasting. 5:2 Diet consists of consuming 500–600 calories for two days of the week and regularly eating for the other five days.

THE 5:2 DIET

DAY 1	DAY 2	DAY 3	DAY 4	DAY 5	DAY 6	DAY 7
Eats normally	Women: 500 calories Men: 600 calories	Eats normally	Eats normally	Women: 500 calories Men: 600 calories	Eats normally	Eats normally

4.4 Eat-and-Stop-and-Eat

Once or twice a week, this Diet requires a full fast for 24 hours. Fitness specialist Brad Pilon made this form of fasting famous, which has been quite known for several years. This leads to a perfect fast of 24 hours if you fast from one dinner to the next dinner the very next day. You've done a perfect 24-hour fast if you end dinner at 8 p.m. Monday and don't feed again before dinner at 8 p.m. Tuesday.

During the short, liquids such as water, coffee, as well and other low-calorie beverages are tolerated, but the solid source of foods is not. You must diet normally during the feeding cycles while you're trying to lose weight. In other words, you can consume as well as you would if you weren't fasting. A complete fast for 24 hours can be challenging for certain citizens, which is a possible disadvantage to this approach. You don't have to go all in straight away, however. It's perfect, to begin with, 14–16 hours, and work your way up. This Diet is a week-long intermittent fasting regimen that includes one of two 24-hour fasts.

4.5 Alternate-Day Fasting

You fast the single day as you practice alternate-day fasting. This approach is available in a variety of forms. During fasting days, some of them make around 500 calories. This technique was used in several of the test-tube trials that showed the health effects of intermittent fasting. A complete fast any other day may seem excessive, so it is not suggested for beginners. This approach can cause you to go to bed many hungry days a week, which is unpleasant and unlikely to be profitable in the long term. Alternate-day fasting entails going without food or consuming just a few hundred calories every second day.

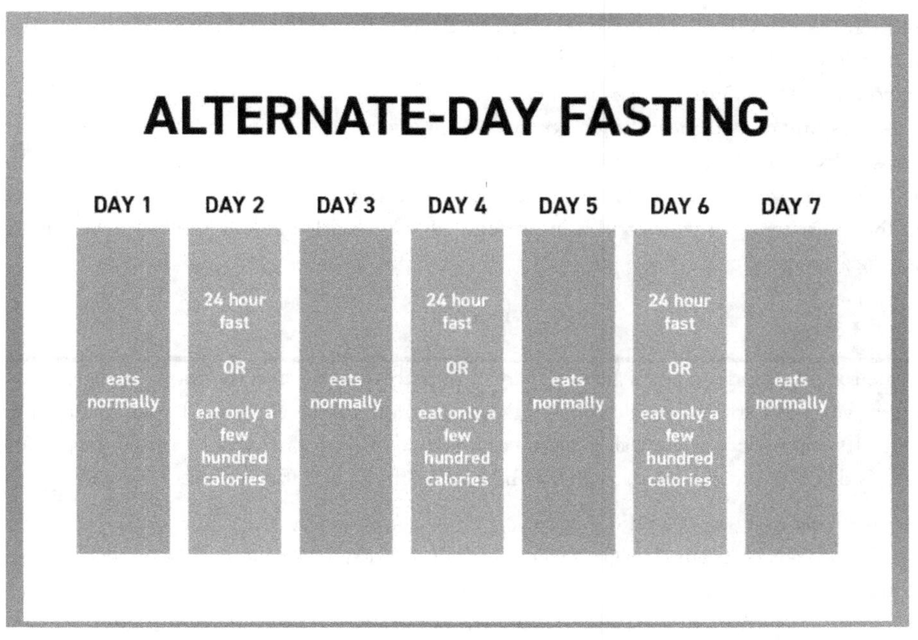

This intermittent fasting is very severe. Throughout a fasting time of 20 hours, this Diet entails consuming very little, normally only a few portions of raw fresh fruits, and vegetables and only enjoying one full meal course at night. Usually, the feeding period is only four hours.

This method of fasting could be more suitable for all those who have tried other forms of intermittent fasting. Advocates for the warrior diet point out that humans are naturally nighttime eaters and feeding at night helps the human body absorb nutrients according to the body's circadian rhythms. Over the four-hour feeding cycle, people can consume plenty of vegetables, proteins, and good fats.

THE WARRIOR DIET

	DAY 1	DAY 2	DAY 3	DAY 4	DAY 5	DAY 6	DAY 7
Midnight – 4 AM – 8 AM – 12 PM	Eating only small amounts of vegetables and fruits	Eating only small amounts of vegetables and fruits	Eating only small amounts of vegetables and fruits	Eating only small amounts of vegetables and fruits	Eating only small amounts of vegetables and fruits	Eating only small amounts of vegetables and fruits	Eating only small amounts of vegetables and fruits
4 PM	Large meal	Large meal	Large meal	Large meal	Large meal	Large meal	Large meal
8 PM – Midnight							

Carbohydrates can also be used. However, it is possible to eat certain items during the fasting time; following the rigid rules for what and when to eat and add to your routine can be difficult. Furthermore, some people find it difficult to consume such a big meal too near to bedtime. There's even a chance that people on this diet won't get enough nutrients like fiber. This will raise cancer incidence and hurt immune and digestive function. Ori Hofmekler, a lifestyle pioneer, popularized this Diet. This warrior diet was among the first popular diets to include an intermittent fasting process. This Diet's dietary habits are like that of the paleo diet since it consists solely of whole, unprocessed foods. This Diet recommends consuming tiny portions of vegetables and fruits during the day and one large dinner at night.

You don't have to stick to a strict intermittent fasting schedule to enjoy any of the advantages. Another choice is to miss meals on occasion, just like when you aren't hungry or when you are too distracted to prepare and eat. It's a fallacy that people must feed every few hours or risk malnutrition or muscle loss. Your body is designed to withstand long stretches of hunger, let alone missing either one or two meals now and then. As a result, if you're not starving one day, miss breakfast and have a nutritious lunch and dinner instead. Alternatively, if you're traveling and can't locate something you want to consume, go on a fast. A random sporadic fast is when you skip one or two meals when you feel like it. During the other meals, make sure you consume nutritious snacks. Another approach to practicing intermittent fasting is to miss one or two meals when you aren't hungry or don't have time to prepare a meal. Intermittent fasting is a weight-loss strategy that works for certain individuals but not for others. Some argue that it might not be as helpful to women as it is to men. It's still not a good idea for individuals who have or are at risk of developing an eating disorder. If you wish to attempt intermittent fasting, remember that the consistency of your food is important. It's impossible to hope to reduce weight and improve your fitness by bingeing on fast food at mealtimes.

Fasting has been done for thousands of years and is a part of numerous faiths and traditions all around the world. Fasting has taken on new meanings in recent years as various varieties of the traditional tradition have emerged. One of the more common fasting types is 16/8 intermittent fasting. Its supporters argue that it is an easy, fast, and long-term way of losing weight and boosting overall health. 16/8 intermittent fasting is discussed in this post, as well as how it functions and if it is correct for you.

WHAT IS 16/8 INTERMITTENT FASTING?

16/8 intermittent fasting entails restricting meal or calorie-containing drinks intake to 8 hours each day and fasting during the next 16 hours. This loop could be replicated as much as you'd prefer, anywhere from once and twice a week to each day, based on your preferences. In past years, 16/8 intermittent fasting has exploded in popularity, particularly among those seeking to reduce weight and burn fat. Some diets have stringent guidelines and rules, but 16/8 intermittent fasting is simple to observe and will yield meaningful results with little effort. It's widely regarded as being less rigid and much more adaptable than most other diet schemes, and it can comfortably blend into almost any lifestyle. 16/8 intermittent fasting is thought to increase blood sugar balance, cognitive activity, and lifespan in addition to promoting weight loss. 16/8 intermittent fasting entails feeding only for eight hours of the day and fasting during the other sixteen. It can help with weight loss, blood sugar control, brain activity, and longevity.

Intermittent fasting (16/8) is easy, healthy, and long-term. To start, choose an 8-hour window and restrict your food consumption to that time frame. Many people choose to consume between midday and.8 p.m., so it allows them to eat a nutritious lunch and dinner, as well as a few treats during the day, while just fasting overnight and skipping breakfast. Others like to consume between the hours of 9 a.m. and 5 p.m., allowing enough time for a nutritious breakfast around 9 a.m., a regular lunch around midday, and a small early dinner and snack between 4 p.m. before beginning their short. You should, therefore, investigate to find the period that works better for you. It's also critical to adhere to healthy whole foods and drinks during your eating cycles to reap the possible health benefits of your Diet. Consuming nutrient-dense foods will help balance out your meals and enable you to enjoy the benefits of this regimen.

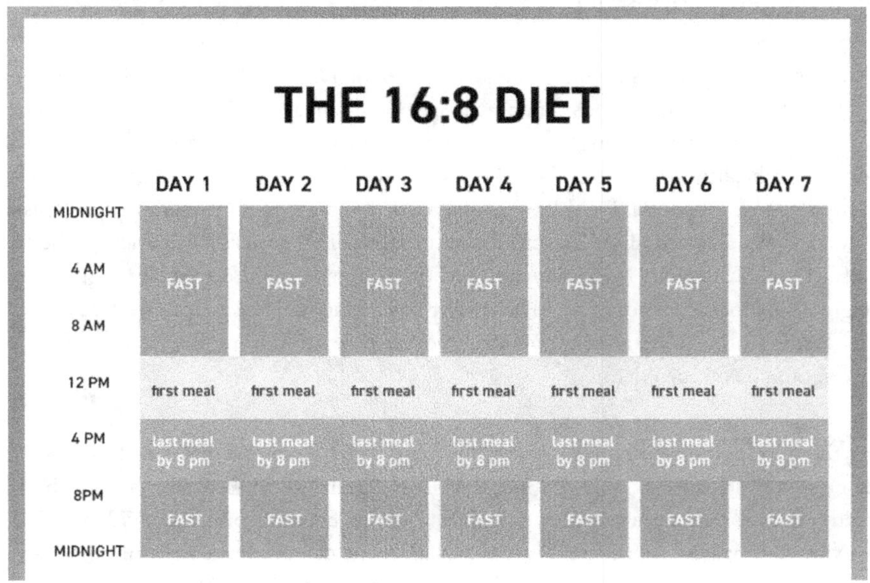

Try to provide a selection of nutritious whole grains in each meal, such as:

- **Veggies:** Broccoli, cauliflower, leafy greens, cucumbers, and tomatoes, etc.
- **Sources of protein:** Meat, poultry, fish, eggs, nuts, legumes, and seeds, etc.
- **Whole grains:** Quinoa, rice, barley, oats, and buckwheat, etc.
- **Fruits:** Apples, bananas, berries, peaches, oranges, pears, etc.
- **Healthy fats:** Avocados, coconut oil, olive oil, etc.

Even when fasting, calorie-free drinks such as water, unsweetened tea, and coffee will help manage your appetite while keeping you hydrated. Overeating or overdoing it on fried food, on the other side, may counteract the benefits of 16/8 intermittent fasting or do more damage than good to your well-being. Choose an 8-hour window and restrict your food consumption to that period to start 16/8 intermittent fasting. During your feeding time, make sure you consume a well-balanced, nutritious diet.

Intermittent fasting (16/8) is a common diet because it is simple to adopt, versatile, and long-term sustainable. It's also useful because it will help you save time and money by reducing a lot of time and cost you spend cooking or food preparation per week.

Intermittent fasting, or 16/8 intermittent fasting, has been linked to a lengthy list of health benefits, including:

- **Increased weight loss**
  Not only does limiting your Diet to several hours per day enable you to burn more calories during the day, but tests suggest that fasting will even improve your appetite and help you lose weight.
- **Improved blood sugar control**
  Intermittent fasting has been shown to lower blood sugar by 3–6% and decrease fasting insulin increase levels to 31%, possibly lowering the risk of diabetes.

- **Enhanced longevity**

    While there is no research in humans, several animal trials have shown that intermittent fasting can help people live longer. 16/8 intermittent fasting is easy, adaptable, and practical. It has been shown in animal and human trials to help people lose weight, reduce blood sugar levels, improve cognitive development, and live longer.

Intermittent fasting (16/8) has many health advantages. However, it still has several disadvantages and might not be suitable for all. Some people may eat more than normal during feeding times to make up for hours spent fasting if they limit their consumption to just eight hours a day. Weight gain, digestion issues, and the growth of poor eating patterns are also possible outcomes. When you first initiate 16/8 intermittent fasting, you can experience short-term negative side effects, including hunger, exhaustion, and fatigue, but these usually fade as you settle into a routine. Furthermore, some literature indicates that intermittent fasting has differing effects on men and women, with animal experiments indicating that it may impair female fertility and reproduction. To assess the impact of intermittent fasting on reproductive health, further human trials are required. In either scenario, begin slowly and pause or contact the doctor if you have any questions or negative symptoms. Regular food restriction may result in fatigue, appetite, increased food consumption, and weight gain. Intermittent fasting has been shown in animal experiments to have various effects on men and women and can also conflict with fertility.

IS 16/8 INTERMITTENT FASTING RIGHT FOR YOU?

When combined with a balanced diet and a supportive lifestyle, 16/8 intermittent fasting can be a sustainable, convenient, and easy way to boost your health. It cannot, though, be considered a replacement for a well-balanced, well-rounded diet abundant in whole foods. Furthermore, even though intermittent fasting does not function for you, you will always remain well. While 16/8 intermittent fasting is deemed safe among most healthy adults, you should consult your doctor before attempting it, particularly if you've any health issues. If you're on certain drugs or have asthma, low blood pressure, or a record of abnormal feeding, this is important. Women who are planning to conceive, nurse, or breastfeed should avoid intermittent fasting. Consult the doctor whether you have any doubts or witness any negative side effects when fasting. 16/8 intermittent fasting entails only feeding for eight hours and fasting for the next sixteen. It can help with weight loss, blood sugar control, brain activity, and longevity. Drink calorie-free drinks like water or unsweetened teas and coffee through the feeding time and follow a balanced diet. Before attempting intermittent fasting, speak with your doctor, particularly if you have any ongoing health problems.

16:8 DIET WEIGHT LOSS

People will consume anything they want during the hours of 10 a.m. and 10 p.m. on this diet. Experts believe that eating between 6 p.m. and 8 p.m. will make people more aware of their appetite signals. Intermittent fasting could be the secret to losing weight and improving your overall health. The study's authors claim that their findings back up previous evidence that time-restricted eating can increase health markers in a variety of ways. Unlike previous studies, this one centered primarily on obese subjects. A total of 23 people were included in the study, with an average age of 45 and 35. The participants were allowed to consume whatever they liked for 12 weeks, but only during the hours of 10 a.m. and 6 p.m. They were instructed to drink only water or calorie-free drinks such as black tea or coffee outside of certain hours.

The plan is known as the "16:8" diet, which corresponds to how many hours you fast and how many hours you consume. Although doctors told them they should eat anything they wanted, they found they used to have a daily calorie cap of about 350 kcal. To put it another way, even though individuals on the 16:8 diet were not told to reduce their food consumption, they wound up eating 350 calories each day on average merely by limiting the period at which they fed. In addition, individuals lost 3% of their body weight and saw a 7% decrease in systolic blood pressure. Fat mass, insulin tolerance, and cholesterol were also assessed, but there was no difference in these indicators between the 16:8 and control groups. People are now more in touch with their eating and appetite signals as they started eating every day, and they quit eating when showed that restricting food intake early in the day reduces the urge to eat later in the day and can boost health, even though the individual does not lose weight.

FOR WHOM 16:8 FASTING ISN'T FOR?

16:8 is something like a dietary modification than a transient diet, according to researchers who were not interested in the research which utilizes the diet from 12 p.m. to 8 p.m. However, experts advise that anyone who is thinking of adopting this behavior should tread carefully. If anyone is on a high-carbohydrate diet until starting this 16:8 diet, their insulin levels would be higher, making them a hypoglycemic nominee (low blood sugar). Diabetics who are uncontrolled or on heavy doses of insulin, as well as patients on diuretic medications, are at risk. Although the 16:8 diet is not completely off-limits for certain individuals, physicians recommend that they seek medical advice to reduce their medication to maintain their lifestyle. While the latest results of the study are encouraging, particularly for people who want to lose weight or reduce their pulse rate without counting calories, it's important to keep in mind that the data set is limited. Another drawback of this technique is that the participants' caloric consumption and commitment to the time were self-reported, implying that the calorie deficit reported in the study might be misleading. Any experts plan to look at the best time for the feeding in the future. People get insulin tolerant increasingly when the day progresses, but they wonder whether having the feeding period before their waking up time will be more effective. Experts often want to see whether reducing the eating window causes people to lose weight or if they stick to the Diet loosely.

Do what you can eat and what you can't

On days when you are not fasting, you can consume about all you want. However, if you want to lose weight and receive the nutrition you need, you can consume nutritious meals and avoid sweets and refined foods. You can consume very little to no food on fasting days. Every Other Day Diet, for example, recommends eating no more than 500 calories on each fast day. Another method, known as the 5:2 Fast Diet, entails consuming five days per week and fasting the remaining two, with women receiving almost 500 calories and men receiving almost 600. That's around a quarter of what you consume on days when you don't find it easy. It's up to you whether you consume certain calories all at once or spread them out over a few micro-meals during the day.

Limitations

It's not easy to go a few days a week without eating any of your calories and focus solely on water, coffee, and tea to keep you satisfied. Despite their brand, you'll need a nutritious meal schedule to consume in balance on your so-called "feast" days. If you want to show progress, you should reward yourself occasionally, but that's about it.

Cooking and shopping

You will manage to prepare and shop as usual if you eat only nutritious foods.

Exercise

It is up to you how much you work out. On your fasting days, though, you won't have much stamina for that. Experts discovered that people who engaged in aerobic activity (such as biking) while fasting on alternating days were able to preserve muscle mass.

Does It Follow Restrictions/Preferences?

You choose what you consume, so it can accommodate dietary restrictions such as vegetarian or veganism, high- or low-carbohydrate diets, fat avoidance, and so on. However, you should be aware that you can experience side effects such as nausea, exhaustion, and headaches.

What Else You Should Know

Cost

Aside from your shopping, there are none. Your food expenses could decrease since you can consume far less two to four days a week.

Support

Several books describe various variants of the general concept of fasting a few days per week. So, while there isn't a specific place to go for help after you've determined which iteration of the proposal applies to you the most, there are lots of options available. On fasting days, most intermittent fasting diets suggest limiting calories to 500-600 calories. In general, more people will find this to be medically better and more convenient than not feeding at all on certain days. To avoid dehydration, consume plenty of water on fasting days.

On days when you don't fast, you'll need to maintain a balanced diet.

Does It Work?

Many studies on intermittent fasting diets have shown that continuing the Diet for several weeks results in at least short-term weight reduction. Can the weight reduction be sustained for a prolonged period? This isn't clear.

Is It Good for Certain Conditions?

According to some studies, this form of Diet may help to reduce asthma symptoms. In addition, several trials, but not all, indicate that the body's usage of insulin is improving. Consult the physicians before attempting intermittent fasting if you have some medical problems. Kids, pregnant mothers, individuals with eating disorders, and certain diabetics are not advised to follow this Diet. For some people, an intermittent fasting diet based on consuming 500-600 calories on an empty stomach can function and be safe.

Figure out caloric needs

When fasting, there are no food limits, but calories must always be counted. People who choose to lose weight must build a calorie shortage, which ensures they gain fewer calories than they expend. Gaining weight necessitates consuming more calories than one expends. Many resources are available to assist an individual in calculating their caloric requirements and determining how many calories they must eat per day to maintain or lose weight. An individual may also seek advice from their doctor or a nutritionist on how many calories they need.

Figure out a meal plan

Making a weekly meal schedule will assist anybody who is attempting to reduce or add weight. An individual who is trying to lose or gain weight can feel that planning their meals each day or week would be beneficial. Meal preparation does not have to be conservative. It considers calorie consumption as well as ensuring that the right foods are used in the Diet. Meal prep has many advantages, including assisting with calorie counting and ensuring that an individual has the requisite ingredients on hand for preparing foods, fast dinners, and snacks.

Make the calories count.

Calories aren't always created equal. Since these fasting techniques do not specify how many calories an individual can ingest when fasting, the nutritional content of the food must be considered. In general, nutrient-dense foods, or food with many nutrients per calorie, should be consumed. Even if an individual does not have to totally avoid fast food, they should still eat it in moderation and concentrate on healthier alternatives to reap the most benefits.

When it comes to misconceptions concerning intermittent fasting, separate reality from fiction; you'll be more able to fast correctly if you have the evidence. And if you fast correctly, you'll be more likely to see the weight loss, consistent energy, and decreased cravings that have rendered intermittent fasting so successful. There is a lot of misinformation out there, unfortunately. Fasting reduces your metabolism, as you've already learned. Fasting causes the muscles to shrivel up, so you shouldn't drink liquids when fasting. Fasting theories, on the other hand, are not founded on fact. Instead, they're built on rumor, speculation, and blind faith in traditional wisdom.

The major intermittent fasting theories will be debunked here. What is the reason for this? As a result, you'll be able to make more educated choices regarding intermittent fasting as an effort to better your fitness. Fasting may be done in a variety of forms. Intermittent fasting is a common eating pattern that includes going without food for a period or severely limiting food intake. A variety of possible health benefits have been attributed to this fasting process, including short-term improvements in human growth hormones and shifts in the expression of genes. Longevity and a reduced incidence of cancer are related to such outcomes. People who fast daily sometimes do so in the hopes of losing weight or living a happier, better existence. Fasting, on the other hand, may be risky if not performed correctly.

5.1 MYTHS ABOUT INTERMITTENT FASTING

When it comes to misconceptions concerning intermittent fasting, separate reality from fiction; you'll be more able to fast correctly if you have the evidence. And if you fast correctly, you'll be more likely to see the weight loss, consistent energy, and decreased cravings that have rendered intermittent fasting so successful. There is a lot of misinformation out there, unfortunately. Fasting reduces your metabolism, as you've already learned. Fasting causes the muscles to shrivel up, so you shouldn't drink liquids when fasting. Fasting theories, on the other hand, are not founded on fact. Instead, they're built on rumor, speculation, and blind faith in traditional wisdom. The major intermittent fasting theories will be debunked here. What is the reason for this? As a result, you'll be able to make more educated choices regarding intermittent fasting as an effort to better your fitness.

FASTING DECREASES YOUR METABOLISM

Some people seem to believe that fasting causes the metabolism to decrease. The fear is that if you resume regular eating habits, you'll add weight like a four-sloth. This is what occurs on calorie-restricted diets, which enable you to consume 50 to 80 % of the total calories the body needs daily for a long time. Your body adjusts to the reduced energy consumption and will do so for years. Non-obese individuals who exercised alternate-day fasting retained a regular metabolism for a maximum of three weeks, even while burning more fat, according to a 2005 report.

YOU SHOULDN'T DRINK WATER WHILE FASTING.

Some religious fasts, such as Ramadan fasting, limit all food and water. Unrelated to this, a host of reports have emerged claiming that no-water diets are beneficial to one's fitness. Due to the diuretic impact of fasting, limiting water can contribute to serious dehydration. That's why, when supervising patients on surgical fasts, doctors pay particular attention to fluid consumption. Electrolytes, including sodium and potassium, which are also vigorously peed out during fasting, are often monitored by doctors. What's the takeaway? During a fast, drink plenty of water and take potassium and sodium supplements if the fast lasts more than 13 or 14 hours.

YOU CAN'T GAIN MUSCLE WHILE FASTING.

Fasting would not seem to be the only way to gain muscle mass. Will you really need to consume protein shakes? Protein is essential, but it is not needed all the time. In one 2019 report, for example, healthy people who fasted 16/8 acquired the same amount of muscle and power as women who ate on a more traditional schedule. Here's the deal: In moments of shortage, the body functions overtime to conserve muscle. When you fast, your body fat (rather than muscle) is used to meet your energy needs. Consider the following scenario: Our forefathers would have become too frail to hunt if they burnt out muscle during a hard.

FASTING MAKES YOU OVERINDULGE

You'll be hungry after a short. Many people believe that this hunger would lead to overeating. The proof, on the other hand, refutes this concern. Ad libitum feeding is a technique used in most fasting trials that allows people to consume as much as they want. They feed to their hearts' content and still lose weight. Most IF protocols would cause you to consume fewer rather than more. As a result of the moderate calorie limit, you'll lose weight gradually without slowing down your metabolism.

Intermittent fasting is all the rage these days. In certain ways, it is sold as being useful to all, all the time. While fasting is generally safe and healthy for most citizens, some groups should avoid it.

Below are some of these organizations:

- Pregnant and nursing women
- Children
- Underweight people

The above groups need more food, not less. Fasting's possible gains are outweighed by the chance of nutritional loss. Those with elevated blood sugar should exercise vigilance as well. Fasting may be beneficial for this group, but medical supervision is needed to avoid extreme hypoglycemia (low blood sugar).

FASTING SAPS YOUR ENERGY.

Food is a source of energy. Would your energy drop if you don't, have it? Yes, eventually. When you fast intermittently, though, the cells switch to a certain pool of energy: body fat. There's enough of it to go around. That's right. Even a thin individual (e.g., 75 kg with 10% body fat) has significant fat reserves to meet energy demands when fasting. Fifteen pounds of fat equals about 60,000 calories of energy if you do the calculations. Many people claim that exercising when fasting gives them more energy. After a big meal, blood is drawn away from tissues and into digestive organs, which makes sense.

YOU CAN'T FOCUS WHILE FASTING.

Consider the last time you were extremely hungry. It wasn't likely your most Zen moment. You should not experience this "hangry" state if you practice intermittent fasting regularly. Your hunger hormones will stabilize once your cells have adapted to using body fat for energy. Burning excess weight also produces ketones, which are small molecules that provide clean, efficient energy to your brain. It's been shown that promoting ketosis increases concentration, interest, and concentration in older adults. It's incredible what this easy and compact eating system will do for the body, brain, and well-being. If you move over the misconceptions of intermittent fasting, you'll see that certain people do better when fasting.

5.2 BEST WAY TO GET STARTED ON A FASTING DIET

Before getting into IF, think of your fitness priorities and take the following steps:

1. **Talk to your primary care doctor.**
   He or she will tell you if this eating style is good for your health. It's important to speak with a healthcare provider if you have concerns about what's best for you. Everybody is different, and depending on the situation, the doctor may have ideas about what you should and shouldn't do.
2. **Choose the best type of IF for you.**
   If you always socialize late at night, for example, 5:2 is likely to be a stronger match than 16:8. Starting with a twelve-hour fast and a twelve-hour feeding window, doctors prescribe gradually increasing to a 14-hour fast and a ten-hour eating window, and eventually to 16:8. Bear in mind, according to the specialist, that the feeding and fasting period is flexible. Few people tend to eat at 10 a.m. and until 6 p.m., while others tend to eat at 12 p.m. and stop at 8 p.m. Figure out what is well for you.
3. **Make sure you have water handy.**
   According to the 2019 report, drinking lots of water throughout the day can help you avoid hunger and absorb fluids that you will usually get from meals.
4. **Limit physical activity**
   Limiting your movements during your fasting cycles is also a smart idea until you recognize how your body will respond.

5.3 HOW TO FAST SAFELY?

Fasting may be done in a variety of forms. Intermittent fasting is a common eating pattern that includes going without food for a period or severely limiting food intake. A variety of possible health benefits have been attributed to this fasting process, including short-term improvements in human growth hormones and shifts in the expression of genes. Longevity and a reduced incidence of cancer are related to such outcomes. People who fast daily sometimes do so in the hopes of losing weight or living a happier, better existence. Fasting, on the other hand, may be risky if not performed correctly.

KEEP FASTING PERIODS SHORT

There is no one-size-fits-all approach to fasting because the length of your fast is entirely up to you. Most of these plans recommend fasting for 8–24 hours. Some participants, on the other hand, prefer to fast for 48 hours or even 72 hours. Fasting over longer amounts of time increases the chances of experiencing complications. Dehydration, moodiness, changes in mood, lightheadedness, appetite, a loss of energy, and inability to concentrate are all symptoms. Shorter fasting times of up to 24 hours are the safest way to prevent these side effects, particularly when you're first starting out. You can obtain medical advice if you plan to extend your fasting time beyond 72 hours. Fasting over longer amounts of time increases the chance of exhaustion, blurry vision, and dehydration. Keep your fasting times brief to reduce your chances.

EAT A SMALL AMOUNT ON FAST DAYS

In principle, fasting entails abstaining from eating and drinking for an amount of time. While you can go without eating on fast days, certain fasting strategies, such as the 5:2 diet, encourage you to eat up to 25% of your daily calorie needs. If you choose to consider fasting, limiting the calories enough that you can only consume limited portions on fast days might be a better choice than going cold turkey. This method can help to alleviate some of the dangers of fasting, such as feeling dizzy, hungry, and distracted. It could even make fasting more manageable, so you won't be as hungry. On fast days, instead of leaving out all calories, eat a limited amount to minimize the chance of adverse effects and hold cravings at bay.

STAY HYDRATED

Mild dehydration may cause nausea, dry mouth, hunger, and headaches, so drinking enough fluid during a fast is critical. To remain hydrated, most health officials prescribe following the 8/8 rule: six eight-ounce glasses of fluid a day. However, although the volume of fluid you need is likely to be in this category, it is highly personal. It's possible to get dehydrated when fasting because food provides around 20–30 percent of the fluid the body requires. Most people tend to consume 8.5–13 cups (2–3 liters) of water during the day while fasting. Nevertheless, your thirst will warn you when you require additional fluids, so pay attention to your body. You can get parched when fasting, and you satisfy some of your everyday fluid requirements with food. To avoid this, pay attention to the details, and how you feel, and drink only when you're thirsty.

GO FOR WALKS OR MEDITATE

It's difficult to avoid eating on fast days, particularly if you're tired and starving. Keeping active is one way to stop unwittingly breaking your fast. Running and meditating are two activities that will help you forget about hunger by not expending too much energy. Every exercise that is relaxing and not too strenuous, on the other hand, can keep the mind occupied. Bathe, reading a novel, or listening to a podcast are all options. Keeping active with low-intensity tasks like walking or meditating will help you stick to your fasting days.

DON'T BREAK FASTS WITH A FEAST.

After a time of restraint, it may be enticing to reward yourself with a large meal. Break your fast with a feast; on the other hand, it can make you feel swollen and exhausted. Furthermore, if you're losing weight, feasting might sabotage your long-term goals by delaying or stopping your losing weight. Eating so many calories after a fast can reduce calorie deficiency, and your final calorie quota affects your weight. The easiest method to break a fast is to eat normally and get to the daily meal schedule. You may feel exhausted and bloated if you consume an unusually big meal during your fast day. Instead, gradually return to regular eating habits.

STOP FASTING IF YOU FEEL UNWELL

You can feel exhausted, hungry, and anxious during a fast, but you should never feel ill. Consider restricting your fast times to 24 hours or less, particularly if you're new to fasting, and keeping a treat on hand just in case you begin to feel sick or sick. If you feel sick or are worried about your welfare, you must immediately avoid fasting. Tiredness or fatigue that prohibits you from performing normal activities, as well as sudden symptoms of nausea and discomfort, are both signals that you can break your fast and pursue medical help. Throughout your fast, you can feel exhausted or irritable, so if you get ill, you can quit fasting instantly.

EAT ENOUGH PROTEIN

Most people begin fasting in terms of weight loss. A calorie deficiency, on the other hand, may result in muscle loss as well as fat loss. Making sure you eat adequate nutrition on the days you eat is one way to prevent muscle failure when fasting. Additionally, if you're just consuming a limited amount of food on fast days, adding any protein might help you manage your appetite. According to several reports, protein consumption of about 30% of a meal's calories will dramatically reduce appetite. As a result, consuming some protein on fast days can help to mitigate some of the negative effects of fasting. Getting enough proteins during your fast will help you avoid muscle failure and control your appetite.

EAT PLENTY OF WHOLE FOODS ON NON-FASTING DAYS

Most citizens fatly do so to better their fitness. Even though fasting requires you to go without food for a period, it is also necessary to live a sustainable lifestyle on days even when you're not fasting. Whole-food diets have been attributed to a variety of health consequences, including a lower incidence of death, cardiac failure, and other chronic conditions. When you feed, use whole foods such as beef, seafood, eggs, grains, fruits, and vegetables to keep your diet balanced. When you're not fasting, eating healthy foods can boost your well-being and help you stay healthy during your fast.

CONSIDER SUPPLEMENTS

You could be missing out on vital nutrients if you are fast daily. This is because consuming fewer calories daily makes it more difficult to satisfy the dietary requirements. People who adopt weight-loss plans are more prone to lacking vital nutrients such as iron, calcium, and b12. As a result, anyone who fasts daily should recommend taking a multivitamin to keep their minds at ease and avoid deficiencies.

However, whole grains are still the greatest source of nutrients. Fasting regularly, particularly when you're in a calorie shortage, will put you at risk for malnutrition. As a result, some individuals opt to take a supplement.

KEEP EXERCISE MILD

Although fasting, certain people feel that they can keep up with their daily workout routine. If you're new to fasting, though, it's better to hold all exercise at a low intensity, particularly at first, to see how you react. Driving, light meditation, soft bending, and household chores are examples of low-intensity workouts. Most specifically, if you're having trouble exercising whilst fasting, pay attention to your body and relax. On fast days, several people can maintain their daily workout schedule. However, if you're new to the fasting diet, it's best to start with light exercise and see how you feel.

5.4 INTERMITTENT FASTING MAY PUT TYPE 2 DIABETES IN REMISSION

Is it possible to push type 2 diabetes into remission by suppressing the eating for a couple of days a week? That's the contentious argument made by researchers in a tiny new report when they fan the flames of a food fad identified as intermittent fasting. However, numerous health experts, including those at the ADA, believe that the technique is risky for people with diabetes, whose bodies are unable to balance their blood sugar through proper nutrition, treatment, and often insulin control. According to the findings of a study, IF, which involves restricting food intake at certain periods of the day or week, helped two middle-aged patients with type 2 diabetes lose some weight, decrease, or eliminate their insulin, and significantly reduce their oral drug. The concern is that we don't approach diabetes as a nutritional issue; instead, we treat it with a slew of medications that never get to the root of the problem.

THE EFFECTS OF INTERMITTENT FASTING ON WEIGHT AND BLOOD SUGAR

Obesity or overweight affects 90% of those with type 2 diabetes. Weight loss is a well-known cure for type 2 diabetes, which involves the bulk of the 30.3 million individuals who have the condition since it aids in the reduction of insulin tolerance and the better absorption of blood glucose. Obesity makes it difficult to monitor diabetes and is a factor contributing to diabetes-related medical problems, according to the CDC. Insulin tolerance, a disease in which the tissues, organs, and liver are unable to consume glucose efficiently, is the characteristic of TD2. This results in high blood sugar and can be treated with medications including Glucophage (metformin) and insulin. Calorie restriction of some form will contribute to losing weight and make blood glucose management simpler. In the absence of glucose from food, intermittent fasting is believed to go a little forward by lowering serum insulin, which causes the body to burn accumulated sugar, or glycogen, as well as fat. Glycogenolysis and lipolysis are two mechanisms that can momentarily lower sugar levels and induce losing weight.

WHY IT'S TOO SOON TO RECOMMEND INTERMITTENT FASTING TO TREAT TYPE 2 DIABETES

One of the causes intermittent fasting is so divisive is the scarcity of large-scale human trials demonstrating its long-term safety and effectiveness. After a year, one report showed that intermittent fasting would not improve type 2 diabetes respondents' blood sugar any more than daily calorie restriction. Intermittent fasting has been shown in mice trials to enhance memory, decrease the risk of disease, and promote weight loss. This isn't necessarily the case for women. Preliminary human trials that have shown promising findings show that the diet warrants more investigation in a broader community for a prolonged period. For the time being, doctors advise patients with diabetes who are taking insulin or sulfonylureas to drop their blood sugar and not to attempt intermittent fasting until consulting with their doctor. Experts believe that while fasting and treating diabetes, medical care is important. If you're taking drugs, you can speak with the doctor, and they'll be the ones to help you.

A LOOK AHEAD AT POSSIBLE INTERMITTENT FASTING RESEARCH

Because of the study's limited sample size and the possible health hazards associated with intermittent fasting, experts claim it's too premature to consider IF as a treatment for diabetes. Physicians are still wary about intermittent fasting's long-term viability. The aim is to achieve long-term weight reduction, and for others, this (intermittent fasting) can be a tough long-term diet habit, which is just what one must do to stay in shape. Despite its common usage in medicine (for example, before colonoscopies) and its use in some religions, like during Ramadan in Islam, experts contend that institutional healthcare finds fasting to be unhealthy. However, something could change in the future. The public's curiosity about fasting has exploded, and scientists are hopeful that this will begin to shift long-held beliefs that fasting is somehow dangerous to our health.

5.5 IF: AN AID IN LOSING WEIGHT

People try intermittent fasting for a variety of reasons, the most common of which is to lose weight. By pushing you to eat fewer calories, intermittent fasting can gradually limit calorie intake. Intermittent fasting will help you lose weight by altering your hormone balance. It increases fat-burning hormone production while also lowering glucose and increasing growth hormone. Short-term intermittent fasting can increase your metabolism by 3–13 % because of hormonal changes. Intermittent fasting helps you lose weight by changing all facets of the caloric continuum, allowing you to eat very little and burn more calories. Intermittent fasting has been shown in studies to be a very effective weight-loss technique. This eating pattern will result in a 3–8% losing weight over 3–24 weeks, according to a 2014 analysis report, which is a large amount in comparison to other weight loss research. People have lost 4–7% of their body composition, showing a substantial loss of unhealthy belly fat that accumulates around the organs and induces illness, according to the report. In another analysis, intermittent fasting was shown to induce less muscle weakness than the more common form of constant calorie restriction. However, keep in mind that the main reason for its appeal is that it helps you to consume fewer calories altogether. You cannot begin to lose much weight if you snack and consume more through your feeding hours. Intermittent fasting can help you eat fewer calories while slightly increasing your metabolism. It's a proven method for losing weight and fat accumulation.

5.6 HEALTH BENEFITS

Intermittent fasting has been studied extensively in both humans and animals. These tests have shown they can help with weight loss along with overall body and brain well-being. It may also assist you in living a longer life.

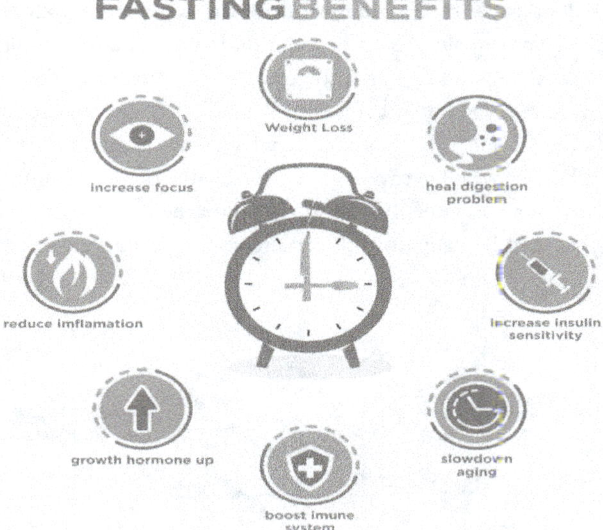

Below are the primary health advantages of intermittent fasting:

- **Weight loss**
  Intermittent fasting, as previously described, will assist you to shed weight and fat accumulation without needing to limit calories actively.

- **Insulin resistance**
  Intermittent fasting will lower blood sugar levels by 3-6 percent and fasting insulin sensitivity levels by 20–31%, reducing insulin resistance and potentially protecting against t2d.

- **Inflammation**
  Inflammation markers, which are a major driver of many chronic diseases, have been shown in several studies to be reduced in several research.

- **Heart health**
  Intermittent fasting has been shown to lower "bad" cholesterol levels, blood triglyceride levels, inflammatory markers, sugar levels, and insulin tolerance, both of which are cardiac disease risk factors.

- **Cancer**
  Intermittent fasting has been shown in animal research to reduce the risk of cancer.

- **Brain Health**
  Intermittent Fasting boosts the brain hormone BDNF, which may help new nerve cells to develop. It may even help to prevent Alzheimer's disease.

- **Anti-aging**
  Intermittent fasting has been shown to increase the lifetime of rats. Fasting rats lived 36-83 percent longer, according to studies. It's important to remember that science is still in its infancy. Most of the experiments were limited, short-term, or animal-based. Many concerns remain unanswered in higher-quality human research. Intermittent fasting has many health advantages for both the body and mind. It will help you lose weight while still lowering the chances of developing type 2 diabetes, cardiac failure, and cancer. It can even assist you in living a longer life.

Good eating is easy, but it can be difficult to sustain. One of the most significant barriers is the amount of time and effort taken to schedule and prepare nutritious meals. Intermittent fasting will make life simpler, so you don't have to prepare, serve, or clean up as many meals as you would otherwise. IF is also very common among the life-hacking community, as it increases your well-being while also facilitating your life. Intermittent fasting has many advantages, one of which is that it allows healthier eating. You'll have less time preparing, cooking, and cleaning up after your meals.

WHO SHOULD BE CAREFUL OR AVOID IT?

Intermittent fasting isn't for everybody. If you're naturally thin or have a background of eating problems, you can check with a doctor before going on a hard. It can be seriously dangerous in these situations.

SHOULD WOMEN FAST?

Intermittent Fasting might not be equally effective for men and women, according to some data. One research found that it reduced insulin sensitivity in males but hindered blood sugar regulation in women, for example. Despite the lack of human research on the topic, studies in rats have shown that IF will trigger female rats to become undernourished, masculine-looking, infertile, and skip periods. Women's menstrual cycles ceased after they began doing IF and returned to usual after they continued their former eating routine, according to empirical studies. Intermittent fasting can be avoided for women for these purposes. They should obey their own set of rules, such as gradually introducing the practice and halting fatly if they have any complications, such as amenorrhea. Consider delaying extended fasting for the time being whether you have pregnancy problems or are planning to conceive. If you're pregnant or breastfeeding, this eating habit is probably not a good one. Fasting is not recommended for those who are underweight and with a history of eating disorders. Intermittent fasting can also be dangerous to certain women, according to some evidence.

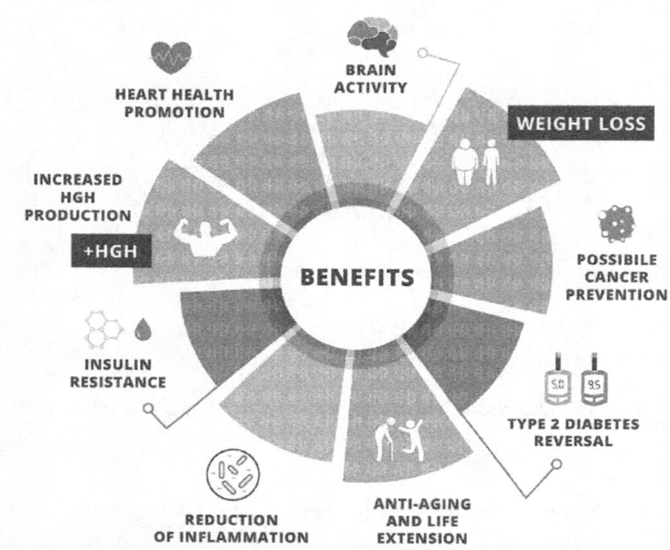

SAFETY AND SIDE EFFECTS

The most common side effect of IF is hunger. You can still feel tired, and the brain may not function as well as it once did. This will only be reversible since the body may need time to adjust to the new dietary pattern. Before attempting intermittent fasting, contact the doctor if you have a medical problem.

This is especially crucial if you:

- Have diabetes
- Have blood sugar balance issues
- Have hypotension.
- Take your medicine as prescribed.
- You're overweight.
- Also had an eating problem in the past.
- You're trying to conceive.
- You've had amenorrhea in the past.
- You're breastfeeding or pregnant.

All things considered, IF has an excellent safety record. If you're safe and well-nourished generally, going without food for a bit isn't risky. Hunger is the most frequent side effect of IF. Fasting cannot be done without first seeing a specialist if you have a medical problem.

Below are responses to some of the most often-asked concerns about intermittent fasting.

1   Can I Drink Liquids during the Fast?

Yes, really. Non-caloric drinks such as water, coffee, and tea are appropriate. Coffee cannot be sweetened. Small quantities of cream or milk may be appropriate. Coffee is particularly helpful during a fast because it suppresses hunger.

2   Isn't It Unhealthy to Skip Breakfast?

No, it's not true. The issue is that most stereotyped breakfast-skippers lead unhealthy lives. The procedure is completely safe if you make sure to consume nutritious options for the remainder of the day.

3   Can I Take Supplements While Fasting?

Yes, really. Bear in mind, though, that certain supplements, such as fat-soluble vitamins, can function best if taken with food.

4   Can I Work Out While Fasting?

Fasted workouts are perfectly acceptable. Before a fasted exercise, certain people consider taking BCAAs.

5   Will Fasting Cause Muscle Loss?

Both weight reduction strategies will result in muscle reduction. That's why it's important to raise weight and consume plenty of protein. Intermittent fasting produces less muscle weakness than normal calorie restriction, according to one report.

6   Will Fasting Slow Down My Metabolism?

No, studies indicate that fasting for a brief period boosts metabolism). Fasting for three or four days, on the other hand, will slow down metabolism.

Re-feeding syndrome is an uncommon consequence of resuming food intake following cycles of starvation or prolonged fasting. It's known as the possibly deadly changes in fluids and salts that malnourished patients may experience. Hypophosphatemia, or extremely poor blood phosphorus levels, and low blood serum phosphorus, calcium, and magnesium levels, are key health indicators. Heart rate disturbances, cardiac failure, breathing complications, convulsions, and coma will also result from these changes. Throughout World War II, the chronically undernourished Americans captured as captives became the first to be diagnosed with this syndrome. It's also been used in the care of long-term anorexia nervosa victims and alcoholics in rehab. Insulin and neutralized hormones, including noradrenaline and cortisol, are reactivated during the re-feeding phase. The passage of large intracellular ions such as phosphate, magnesium, calcium, and potassium through our cells is caused by this. However, owing to the loss of our body's total reserves, this becomes unnecessary, and we end up having very little of such ions in our blood.

Below are the key signs of this syndrome:

- Tiredness
- Weakness
- Perplexity
- Breathing problems or inability to breathe
- High blood pressure
- Seizures
- Heart arrhythmias
- Heart attack
- Coma
- Death

These signs usually occur two to four days after you begin refeeding.

ARE YOU AT RISK OF REFEEDING SYNDROME?

Rather than being undernourished, most of them are currently over nourished. However, this would not negate the need for vigilance. Certain types of people are more likely than others to have refeeding syndrome:

- The BMI (body mass index) is around 18.5.
- You've lost more than 10% of the body mass in the past six months due to unintentional weight loss.
- You've fasted for five days or so, drinking just liquids.
- You have lower-than-normal amounts of arsenic, potassium, calcium, or magnesium in the serum.

- You have a background of drinking or becoming an addict.
- You suffer from anorexia nervosa.
- Use insulin, blood thinners, naproxen, or are doing chemotherapy.

When you do break your hard, there are a few things you can do to reduce your chances of having refeeding issues:

- Avoid breaking the fast with a high-carbohydrate meal; instead, go for low-carb, high-fat options. Avoid high-insulin and high-blood-sugar foods.
- Drink mineral water to drink fluids during your fast.
- A tablespoon of natural salts, such as Himalayan salt, may be added to the diet many times during the day.
- If you're planning a prolonged early, talk to the doctor first.

When fasting for fewer than 36 hours, you don't have to be concerned with what to eat once you end your fast. Stick with low-carb, high-fat foods, such as some of the Diet Doctor's dishes that sound enticing. Try not to overeat. When you start feeding, fasting is not an opportunity to indulge yourself. If you're trying to fast for a prolonged period, think about how you'll break it. Resuming food with a tiny lunch and eating steadily is a good idea. Start with a bone broth or any psyllium husk dissolved in water. Eat a small new tomato, then cucumber salad, and stick to light proteins like tuna or chicken that are around the size of your hand or a card game.

Chapter 6.

28-Day Meal Plan

DAY	BREAKFAST	LUNCH	SNACK	DINNER
1	Almond Butter and Banana Chia Pudding	Mediterranean Chickpea Salad	Apple Slices with Peanut Butter	Grilled Salmon with Asparagus
2	Greek Yogurt with Mixed Berries	Quinoa Tabbouleh	Carrot Sticks with Hummus	Chicken Stir-Fry with Vegetables
3	Overnight Oats with Mango	Lentil Soup	Almonds and Dark Chocolate	Baked Cod with Roasted Sweet Potatoes
4	Spinach and Feta Omelet	Avocado Chicken Salad	Greek Yogurt and Honey	Vegetable Curry with Brown Rice
5	Smoothie Bowl with Nuts and Seeds	Tuna Salad Stuffed Avocados	Cottage Cheese with Pineapple	Eggplant Parmesan
6	Avocado Toast with Egg	Turkey and Spinach Wrap	Mixed Nuts	Shrimp and Broccoli Stir-Fry
7	Berry and Banana Smoothie	Caprese Salad with Grilled Chicken	Fresh Fruit Salad	Zucchini Noodles with Pesto

DAY	BREAKFAST	LUNCH	SNACK	DINNER
8	Whole Grain Toast with Almond Butter	Sweet Potato and Black Bean Burrito	Rice Cakes with Avocado	Lemon Herb Roasted Chicken
9	Cottage Cheese with Fresh Berries	Caesar Salad with Salmon	Edamame	Quinoa Stuffed Bell Peppers
10	Scrambled Eggs with Spinach and Feta	Chicken Caesar Wrap	Dark Chocolate and Berries	Fish Tacos with Cabbage Slaw
11	Protein Pancakes	Vegetable Stir-Fry with Tofu	Hummus and Veggie Sticks	Beef and Vegetable Skewers
12	Chia Seed Pudding with Kiwi	Turkey Cobb Salad	Greek Yogurt with Cinnamon	Spaghetti Squash with Tomato Sauce
13	Oatmeal with Apples and Cinnamon	Grilled Veggie and Hummus Flatbread	Protein Shake	Chicken and Vegetable Soup
14	Mixed Berry Parfait	Shrimp Avocado Salad	Apple with Almond Butter	Turkey Chili

15	Avocado and Cottage Cheese Toast	Roasted Beet and Goat Cheese Salad	Sliced Cucumber with Lime and Salt	Lemon Garlic Tilapia with Steamed Broccoli
16	Berry Protein Smoothie	Chickpea and Cucumber Sandwich	Peach Slices with Cottage Cheese	Vegetable Lasagna
17	Whole Wheat Pancakes with Blueberries	Lentil and Avocado Salad	Celery Sticks with Almond Butter	Stuffed Acorn Squash
18	Yogurt with Granola and Honey	Tofu Stir-Fry with Broccoli and Peppers	Mixed Berries	Grilled Chicken with Quinoa and Green Beans
19	Scrambled Tofu with Spinach and Tomatoes	Chicken and Avocado Wrap	Nuts and Seeds Mix	Fish Fillet with Mixed Vegetable Salad
20	Muesli with Skim Milk	Beef and Arugula Salad	Dark Chocolate Square	Roasted Butternut Squash Risotto
21	Banana and Almond Milk Smoothie	Turkey Lettuce Wraps	Granola Bar	Pizza with Cauliflower Crust

22	Omelet with Mushrooms and Onions	Salmon Salad with Mixed Greens	Yogurt with Pumpkin Seeds	Stir-Fried Tofu with Brown Rice and Veggies
23	Cottage Cheese with Honey and Walnuts	Grilled Cheese with Tomato Soup	Fresh Pineapple Chunks	Beef Stir-Fry with Bell Peppers and Snow Peas
24	Fruit Salad with Chia Seeds	Quinoa Salad with Roasted Vegetables	Hard-Boiled Egg	Chicken Fajitas with Whole Wheat Tortillas
25	Overnight Oats with Peanut Butter	Tuna Salad on Whole Grain Bread	Apple and Peanut Butter	Baked Sweet Potato with Grilled Vegetables
26	Spinach and Banana Smoothie	Caesar Salad with Grilled Shrimp	Cottage Cheese with Sliced Peaches	Pan-Seared Salmon with Asparagus and Quinoa
27	English Muffin with Poached Egg and Avocado	Soba Noodles with Peanut Sauce	Trail Mix	Zucchini Lasagna
28	Nut Butter and Jelly Oatmeal	Soba Noodle Salad with Edamame	Cheese and Whole Grain Crackers	Grilled Steak with Roasted Vegetables

1) ALMOND BUTTER AND BANANA CHIA PUDDING

Preparation Time: 10 minutes	**Cooking Time:** 0 minutes	**Servings:** 2

INGREDIENTS:

2 tablespoons chia seeds 1/2 cup almond milk (unsweetened) 1 tablespoon almond butter	1 ripe banana, mashed 1/2 teaspoon vanilla extract A pinch of cinnamon (optional)	A few slices of banana and a sprinkle of chopped almonds, for topping

INSTRUCTIONS:

1. In a bowl, combine chia seeds, almond milk, almond butter, mashed banana, and vanilla extract. Add a pinch of cinnamon for extra flavor if desired. Mix well until all the ingredients are fully combined.
2. Cover the mixture and refrigerate overnight, allowing the chia seeds to swell and the pudding to thicken.
3. Before serving, give the pudding a good stir. If it's too thick, you can adjust the consistency by adding a little more almond milk.
4. Serve the pudding in bowls, topped with banana slices, and chopped almonds for added texture and flavor.

NUTRITIONAL VALUES (PER SERVING):

✓ Calories: 280 ✓ Protein: 6g	✓ Fat: 15g ✓ Carbohydrates: 30g	✓ Fiber: 10g

PREPARATION TIPS:

- For a smoother texture, blend the mixture before refrigerating.
- Toasting the almonds lightly will enhance their flavor and add a delightful crunch.

SHOPPING TIPS:

- Choose ripe bananas for natural sweetness and a creamy texture.
- Opt for natural, unsweetened almond butter to avoid added sugars and oils.

ALTERNATIVE VARIATIONS:

- Swap almond butter for peanut or cashew butter for a different flavor.
- Add a layer of fresh berries at the bottom of the bowl before adding the pudding for an extra fruit serving.

2) ALMOND BUTTER OATMEAL WITH BERRIES

Preparation Time: 5 minutes	**Cooking Time:** 10 minutes	**Servings:** 2

INGREDIENTS:

1 cup rolled oats 2 cups water or almond milk 2 tablespoons almond butter	1 cup mixed berries (blueberries, strawberries, raspberries) 1 tablespoon chia seeds	1 tablespoon honey or maple syrup (optional) A pinch of salt

INSTRUCTIONS:

1. In a saucepan, bring water or almond milk to a boil. Add the oats and a pinch of salt, then reduce the heat to a simmer.
2. Cook the oats, stirring occasionally, until they are soft and have absorbed the liquid, about 5 minutes.
3. Stir in the almond butter until well combined. If using, sweeten with honey or maple syrup.
4. Divide the oatmeal into bowls and top with mixed berries and a sprinkle of chia seeds.
5. Serve warm for a nutritious and satisfying breakfast.

NUTRITIONAL VALUES (PER SERVING):

✓ Calories: 320 ✓ Protein: 10g	✓ Fat: 14g ✓ Carbohydrates: 44g	✓ Fiber: 9g

PREPARATION TIPS:

- For a smoother texture, add the almond butter to the oatmeal while it's cooking.

SHOPPING TIPS:

- Opt for organic, old-fashioned rolled oats for their texture and nutritional benefits. Choose fresh or frozen berries depending on availability.

ALTERNATIVE VARIATIONS:

- Swap almond butter with peanut or cashew butter for a different flavor profile. Add nuts or seeds for extra crunch and protein.

3) AVOCADO AND COTTAGE CHEESE TOAST

<table>
<tr><td>Preparation Time: 5 minutes</td><td>Cooking Time: 2 minutes</td><td>Servings: 2</td></tr>
</table>

INGREDIENTS:

2 slices whole grain bread 1 ripe avocado, sliced 1/2 cup cottage cheese	Salt and pepper to taste Red pepper flakes (optional)	Fresh herbs for garnish (optional, such as chives or parsley)

INSTRUCTIONS:

1. Toast the whole grain bread slices until golden and crispy.
2. Spread the cottage cheese evenly over the toasted bread slices.
3. Arrange the avocado slices on top of the cottage cheese. Season with salt and pepper. Add red pepper flakes if you like a bit of heat.
4. Garnish with fresh herbs if desired for an added burst of flavor and color.

NUTRITIONAL VALUES (PER SERVING):

✓ Calories: Approximately 300 ✓ Protein: 12g	✓ Fat: 15g ✓ Carbohydrates: 32g	✓ Fiber: 8g

PREPARATION TIPS:

- For added texture and nutrition, sprinkle some pumpkin seeds or sunflower seeds on top of the avocado.
- Lightly drizzling the avocado with lemon juice not only adds a zesty flavor but also helps prevent browning.

SHOPPING TIPS:

- Choose avocados that yield to gentle pressure for the best creaminess. Avoid those with dark spots or bruises.
- Look for cottage cheese with live cultures for an extra probiotic boost.

ALTERNATIVE VARIATIONS:

- For a dairy-free version, substitute cottage cheese with a dairy-free spread such as almond ricotta or cashew cream cheese.
- Add sliced tomatoes or cucumbers for an extra layer of freshness and crunch.

4) *AVOCADO AND EGG SPINACH SALAD*

<table>
<tr><td>Preparation Time: 10 minutes</td><td>Cooking Time: 5 minutes</td><td>Servings: 2</td></tr>
</table>

INGREDIENTS:

2 eggs, boiled and sliced 1 ripe avocado, sliced 2 cups fresh spinach leaves	1/4 red onion, thinly sliced 2 tablespoons olive oil 1 tablespoon balsamic vinegar	Salt and pepper to taste

INSTRUCTIONS:

1. On two plates, lay out the spinach leaves.
2. Top with the avocado slices, boiled egg slices, and red onion.
3. Whisk olive oil and balsamic vinegar in a bowl, then drizzle over the salads.
4. Season with salt and pepper as desired and serve.

NUTRITIONAL VALUES (PER SERVING):

✓ Calories: 290 ✓ Protein: 8g	✓ Fat: 25g ✓ Carbohydrates: 12g	✓ Fiber: 7g

PREPARATION TIPS:

- Add toasted nuts or seeds for an additional crunch and nutritional boost.

SHOPPING TIPS:

- Choose avocados that are slightly soft to the touch for peak ripeness.

ALTERNATIVE VARIATIONS:

- Try using arugula or kale in place of spinach for a different taste and texture.

5) *AVOCADO TOAST WITH EGG*

<table>
<tr><td>Preparation Time: 5 minutes</td><td>Cooking Time: 5 minutes</td><td>Servings: 2</td></tr>
</table>

INGREDIENTS:

2 slices whole grain bread 1 ripe avocado	2 eggs Salt and pepper to taste	Red pepper flakes (optional) Olive oil (for the egg)

INSTRUCTIONS:

1. Toast the whole-grain bread to your liking.
2. Mash the avocado in a bowl and season with salt and pepper. Spread the mashed avocado evenly onto the toasted bread.
3. Heat a small amount of olive oil in a pan over medium heat. Crack the eggs into the pan and cook to your preference (sunny side up recommended).
4. Place the cooked egg on top of the avocado toast. Season with salt, pepper, and red pepper flakes if desired.

NUTRITIONAL VALUES (PER SERVING):

✓ Calories: 350 ✓ Protein: 12g	✓ Fat: 20g ✓ Carbohydrates: 30g	✓ Fiber: 8g

PREPARATION TIPS:

- For an extra protein boost, consider adding smoked salmon or turkey slices on top of the avocado before adding the egg.
- Use a fork to create small wells in the avocado spread to help keep the egg in place.

SHOPPING TIPS:

- Choose avocados that are slightly soft to the touch for the perfect ripeness.
- Opt for bread that's high in fiber and whole grains for added nutritional benefits.

ALTERNATIVE VARIATIONS:

- For a vegan option, replace the egg with tofu scramble or sliced tomatoes.

6) BANANA AND ALMOND MILK SMOOTHIE

Preparation Time: 5 minutes	**Cooking Time:** 0 minutes	**Servings:** 2

INGREDIENTS:

2 ripe bananas 2 cups almond milk 1 tablespoon almond butter:	(Optional, for added richness) A pinch of cinnamon: (Optional, for flavor)	Ice cubes: (Optional, for a colder smoothie)

INSTRUCTIONS:

1. Place the bananas, almond milk, and almond butter (if using) in a blender.
2. Add a pinch of cinnamon for a hint of spice.
3. Blend until smooth. Add ice cubes if you prefer a chilled smoothie.
4. Pour into glasses and enjoy immediately.

NUTRITIONAL VALUES (PER SERVING):

✓ Calories: Approximately 180 ✓ Protein: 3g	✓ Fat: 4g ✓ Carbohydrates: 35g	✓ Fiber: 4g

PREPARATION TIPS:

- For an extra protein boost, add a scoop of your favorite protein powder.
- Freeze the bananas ahead of time for an extra thick and creamy smoothie texture.

SHOPPING TIPS:

- Choose unsweetened almond milk to control the sweetness of your smoothie.
- Ripe bananas provide natural sweetness, reducing the need for added sugars.

ALTERNATIVE VARIATIONS:

- Swap almond milk for any other plant-based milk you prefer.
- Add a handful of spinach for a green smoothie version without altering the taste much.

7) BERRY AND BANANA SMOOTHIE

Preparation Time: 5 minutes	**Cooking Time:** 0 minutes	**Servings:** 2

INGREDIENTS:

1 ripe banana 1 cup mixed berries (such as strawberries, blueberries, raspberries, and blackberries), fresh or frozen	1 cup Greek yogurt (plain or vanilla) 1/2 cup almond milk (or any milk of your choice)	1 tablespoon honey or maple syrup (optional, for added sweetness) Ice cubes (optional, for a thicker and colder smoothie)

INSTRUCTIONS:

1. In a blender, combine the banana, mixed berries, Greek yogurt, and almond milk.
2. Add honey or maple syrup if you prefer a sweeter taste.
3. If you're using fresh fruits and prefer a colder smoothie, add a few ice cubes.
4. Blend on high until smooth and creamy. If the smoothie is too thick, add a little more milk to reach your desired consistency.
5. Pour the smoothie into glasses and serve immediately. Enjoy the burst of energy and flavors!

NUTRITIONAL VALUES (PER SERVING):

✓ Calories: 220 ✓ Protein: 12g	✓ Fat: 3g ✓ Carbohydrates: 40g	✓ Fiber: 5g

PREPARATION TIPS:

- Using frozen berries will give the smoothie a cold and refreshing texture without the need for ice.
- For an extra protein boost, add a scoop of your favorite protein powder.

SHOPPING TIPS:

- When buying berries, look for ones that are bright, firm, and free of mold. If opting for frozen berries, check that they're free from added sugars.
- Choose a high-quality Greek yogurt for added protein and a creamy texture.

ALTERNATIVE VARIATIONS:

- Swap Greek yogurt with a plant-based yogurt to make this smoothie vegan.
- Add a handful of spinach or kale for an extra serving of vegetables without altering the fruity taste significantly.

8) BERRY PROTEIN SMOOTHIE

Preparation Time: 5 minutes	**Cooking Time:** 0 minutes	**Servings:** 2

INGREDIENTS:

1 cup mixed berries (fresh or frozen) 1 banana, for added sweetness and texture	1 scoop protein powder (preferably vanilla or berry flavored) 1 cup almond milk (or any milk of your choice)	Ice cubes (optional, for a colder smoothie)

INSTRUCTIONS:

1. Place the mixed berries, banana, protein powder, and almond milk in a blender. Add ice cubes if you prefer a chilled smoothie.
2. Blend on high until smooth and creamy. Add more milk if needed to reach your desired consistency.
3. Taste and adjust the sweetness by adding a little honey or maple syrup if desired.
4. Pour into glasses and serve immediately. Enjoy the burst of energy and flavor!

NUTRITIONAL VALUES (PER SERVING):

✓ Calories: Approximately 250 ✓ Protein: 20g	✓ Fat: 3g ✓ Carbohydrates: 35g	✓ Fiber: 5g

PREPARATION TIPS:

- For an extra fiber boost, add a tablespoon of flaxseeds or chia seeds to the blender before mixing.
- If using frozen berries, you can omit the ice cubes to avoid diluting the smoothie.

SHOPPING TIPS:

- Select a protein powder that complements the natural flavors of the berries for the best taste experience.
- When available, opt for organic berries to reduce exposure to pesticides.

ALTERNATIVE VARIATIONS:

- Swap out almond milk with coconut water for a lighter, hydrating version.
- Mix and match your berries based on seasonal availability and personal preference for varied flavors.

9) CHIA SEED PUDDING WITH KIWI

Preparation Time: 10 minutes	**Cooking Time:** 0 minutes	**Servings:** 2

INGREDIENTS:

1/4 cup chia seeds 1 cup coconut milk (or any milk of choice)	1 tablespoon maple syrup or honey 1 teaspoon vanilla extract 2 kiwis, peeled and sliced	A few mint leaves for garnish (optional)

INSTRUCTIONS:

1. In a mixing bowl, combine chia seeds, coconut milk, maple syrup (or honey), and vanilla extract. Stir well until the mixture is homogenous.
2. Cover the bowl and refrigerate overnight, allowing the chia seeds to absorb the liquid and swell up, forming a pudding-like consistency.
3. Before serving, give the chia pudding a good stir. If it's too thick, you can adjust the consistency by adding a little more milk.
4. Divide the pudding into serving bowls or glasses and top with sliced kiwi. Garnish with mint leaves if desired.

NUTRITIONAL VALUES (PER SERVING):

✓ Calories: 300 ✓ Protein: 5g	✓ Fat: 20g ✓ Carbohydrates: 25g	✓ Fiber: 10g

PREPARATION TIPS:

- For a smoother pudding, blend the mixture before chilling.
- You can prepare the pudding in individual jars for an easy grab-and-go breakfast option.

SHOPPING TIPS:

- Choose ripe kiwis for the best flavor and sweetness.
- If using canned coconut milk, opt for the light version for a lower-calorie option.

ALTERNATIVE VARIATIONS:

- Substitute kiwi with any other fruit of your choice, such as berries, mango, or peach.
- For added texture and crunch, top with granola or nuts before serving.

10) CHIA SEED PUDDING WITH MIXED BERRIES

Preparation Time: 10 minutes	**Cooking Time:** 0 minutes	**Servings:** 2

INGREDIENTS:

1/4 cup chia seeds 1 cup unsweetened almond milk	1 tablespoon maple syrup or honey (optional) 1/2 teaspoon vanilla extract	1 cup mixed berries (Blueberries, strawberries, raspberries) A pinch of salt

INSTRUCTIONS:

1.In a bowl, mix chia seeds, almond milk, maple syrup (or honey), vanilla extract, and a pinch of salt. Stir well until combined.
2.Cover and refrigerate overnight, or at least 6 hours, until it has a pudding-like consistency.
3.Before serving, stir the pudding once more, and if it's too thick, adjust by adding a little more almond milk.
4.Serve in bowls, topped with mixed berries.

NUTRITIONAL VALUES (PER SERVING):

✓ Calories: 200	✓ Fat: 9g	✓ Fiber: 10g
✓ Protein: 5g	✓ Carbohydrates: 24g	

PREPARATION TIPS:

• For an extra smooth pudding, blend the mixture before refrigerating.

SHOPPING TIPS:

• Pick up fresh, seasonal berries for the best flavor and nutritional value. Frozen berries can also be a great alternative.

ALTERNATIVE VARIATIONS:

• Experiment with different milks for varied flavors or add nut butter for an extra protein and flavor boost.

11) COTTAGE CHEESE WITH FRESH BERRIES

Preparation Time: 5 minutes	Cooking Time: 0 minutes	Servings: 2

INGREDIENTS:

1 cup cottage cheese	(Strawberries, blueberries, raspberries)	2 tablespoons chopped nuts
1/2 cup mixed fresh berries	1 tablespoon honey (optional)	(Almonds, walnuts, or pecans; optional)

INSTRUCTIONS:

1.Divide the cottage cheese between two bowls.
2.Top each bowl with a generous portion of mixed fresh berries.
3.Drizzle honey over the berries and cottage cheese for a touch of sweetness, if desired.
4.Sprinkle chopped nuts on top for added texture and a nutty flavor, if using.

NUTRITIONAL VALUES (PER SERVING):

✓ Calories: 200	✓ Fat: 8g (varies with the type of nuts used)	✓ Fiber: 2g
✓ Protein: 14g	✓ Carbohydrates: 18g	

PREPARATION TIPS:

• For the best flavor and nutritional benefits, choose fresh, in-season berries.

• If you prefer a smoother texture, blend the cottage cheese until creamy before adding the toppings.

SHOPPING TIPS:

• Look for low-fat or full-fat cottage cheese based on your dietary preferences.

• Organic berries are recommended to reduce exposure to pesticides.

ALTERNATIVE VARIATIONS:

• Substitute berries with other fruits like sliced peaches, mango, or kiwi for variety.

• For a dairy-free version, use a plant-based yogurt alternative.

12) COTTAGE CHEESE WITH HONEY AND WALNUTS

Preparation Time: 5 minutes	Cooking Time: 0 minutes	Servings: 2

INGREDIENTS:

1 cup cottage cheese	2 tablespoons honey	Fresh fruit for topping (optional, such as
2 tablespoons walnuts, chopped		sliced strawberries or peaches)

INSTRUCTIONS:

1.Divide the cottage cheese between two bowls.
2.Sprinkle chopped walnuts over the cottage cheese.
3.Drizzle honey over the top.
4.Add fresh fruit toppings if desired for additional flavor and nutrients.

NUTRITIONAL VALUES (PER SERVING):

✓ Calories: Approximately 220	✓ Fat: 10g	✓ Fiber: 0g
✓ Protein: 14g	✓ Carbohydrates: 18g	

PREPARATION TIPS:

• For added texture and flavor, lightly toast the walnuts before adding them to the dish.

• Adjust the amount of honey to suit your taste preferences.

SHOPPING TIPS:

• Look for full-fat cottage cheese for a creamier texture and richer flavor.

• Raw, local honey not only tastes better but also provides more health benefits.

ALTERNATIVE VARIATIONS:

- Substitute walnuts with almonds, pecans, or any other nuts of your choice.
- Mix in a pinch of cinnamon or vanilla extract to the cottage cheese for an extra layer of flavor.

13) ENGLISH MUFFIN WITH POACHED EGG AND AVOCADO

Preparation Time: 10 minutes	**Cooking Time:** 5 minutes	**Servings:** 2

INGREDIENTS:

2 English muffins, split and toasted 1 ripe avocado, mashed	2 eggs, poached Salt and pepper to taste	Red pepper flakes or paprika (optional, for garnish)

INSTRUCTIONS:

1. Toast the English muffins until golden and crispy.
2. Spread the mashed avocado onto each half of the English muffins.
3. Top each half with a poached egg. Season with salt and pepper, adding red pepper flakes or paprika if desired.
4. Serve immediately, savoring the blend of textures and flavors.

NUTRITIONAL VALUES (PER SERVING):

✓ Calories: 350 ✓ Protein: 15g	✓ Fat: 20g ✓ Carbohydrates: 30g	✓ Fiber: 7g

PREPARATION TIPS:

- To poach the eggs, use a simmering pot of water with a splash of vinegar, swirling the water before adding the eggs for a more cohesive white.
- Experiment with additional toppings like sautéed spinach or sliced tomatoes for extra nutrients and flavors.

SHOPPING TIPS:

- Look for whole-grain English muffins to add extra fiber to your breakfast.
- Avocados should be slightly soft to the touch; buying them a few days in advance allows them to ripen to perfection.

ALTERNATIVE VARIATIONS:

- For a gluten-free option, substitute the English muffin with a gluten-free version or use sliced toasted sweet potato.
- Add smoked salmon or turkey bacon for an extra protein boost and a smoky flavor.

14) FRUIT SALAD WITH CHIA SEEDS

Preparation Time: 10 minutes	**Cooking Time:** 0 minutes	**Servings:** 2

INGREDIENTS:

2 cups mixed fresh fruit (such as berries, kiwi, mango, and apple) 2 tablespoons chia seeds	Juice of 1 lime Mint leaves for garnish (optional)	Honey or maple syrup for sweetness (optional)

INSTRUCTIONS:

1. In a large bowl, combine the mixed fresh fruit.
2. Sprinkle chia seeds over the fruit and add lime juice. Gently toss to combine.
3. Let the salad sit for about 5 minutes to allow the chia seeds to begin to gel.
4. Serve in bowls, garnished with mint leaves, and drizzled with honey or maple syrup if desired.

NUTRITIONAL VALUES (PER SERVING):

✓ Calories: Approximately 150 ✓ Protein: 3g	✓ Fat: 4g ✓ Carbohydrates: 27g	✓ Fiber: 6g

PREPARATION TIPS:

- Cut the fruit into uniform pieces for a balanced mix of flavors in every bite.
- The lime juice not only adds flavor but also helps prevent the fruit from browning.

SHOPPING TIPS:

- Choose a variety of colors and textures in your fruits to make the salad more appealing and nutritious.
- Organic fruits are preferred for their lower pesticide levels and potentially higher nutrient content.

ALTERNATIVE VARIATIONS:

- Sprinkle granola on top for an added crunch.
- For a tropical twist, add a splash of coconut water to the salad.

15) GREEK YOGURT WITH MIXED BERRIES

Preparation Time: 5 minutes	**Cooking Time:** 0 minutes	**Servings:** 2

INGREDIENTS:

1 cup Greek yogurt (unsweetened) 1/2 cup mixed berries (strawberries, blueberries, raspberries, blackberries)	2 teaspoons honey (optional) A sprinkle of granola (optional) A few mint leaves for garnish (optional)

INSTRUCTIONS:

1.Divide the Greek yogurt between two bowls.
2.Top with an even layer of mixed berries.
3.Drizzle with honey for a touch of sweetness, if desired.
4.Add a sprinkle of granola for added texture and flavor, if using.
5.Garnish with mint leaves to enhance the freshness of the dish.

NUTRITIONAL VALUES (PER SERVING):

✓ Calories: 150 (without granola) ✓ Protein: 20g	✓ Fat: 4g ✓ Carbohydrates: 12g (without honey)	✓ Fiber: 2g

PREPARATION TIPS:

- For the best flavor and nutritional value, use fresh, in-season berries.
- If you prefer a thinner yogurt consistency, stir in a little milk or water before adding the toppings.

SHOPPING TIPS:

- Opt for full-fat Greek yogurt for a richer texture and better satiety.
- Choose organic berries, when possible, to reduce exposure to pesticides.

ALTERNATIVE VARIATIONS:

- Swap Greek yogurt for a dairy-free alternative like coconut yogurt to cater to dietary restrictions or preferences.

16) MIXED BERRY PARFAIT

Preparation Time: 10 minutes	**Cooking Time:** 0 minutes	**Servings:** 2

INGREDIENTS:

1 cup Greek yogurt (plain or vanilla) 1 cup mixed berries (strawberries, blueberries, raspberries, blackberries)	1/2 cup granola Honey or maple syrup (optional for sweetness)	Mint leaves for garnish (optional)

INSTRUCTIONS:

1.If using larger berries like strawberries, slice them into smaller pieces for easier layering.
2.In serving glasses or bowls, start by layering a spoonful of Greek yogurt at the bottom.
3.Add a layer of mixed berries on top of the yogurt.
4.Sprinkle a layer of granola over the berries.
5.Repeat the layers until the glasses or bowls are filled, finishing with a layer of berries on top.
6.Drizzle with a little honey or maple syrup for added sweetness, if desired.
7.Garnish with mint leaves for a refreshing touch.

NUTRITIONAL VALUES (PER SERVING):

✓ Calories: 280 ✓ Protein: 15g	✓ Fat: 6g ✓ Carbohydrates: 44g	✓ Fiber: 5g

PREPARATION TIPS:

- For a vegan option, use plant-based yogurt alternatives such as coconut yogurt or almond yogurt.
- Making this parfait the night before can save time in the morning and allow the flavors to meld beautifully.

SHOPPING TIPS:

- Choose fresh, organic berries for the best taste and nutritional value. Frozen berries can also work well if fresh ones are not available.
- Look for low-sugar granola to keep the parfait healthy and not overly sweet.

ALTERNATIVE VARIATIONS:

- Mix in a scoop of protein powder with the yogurt for an extra protein boost.
- Substitute granola with nuts or seeds for a different texture.

17) MUESLI WITH SKIM MILK

Preparation Time: 5 minutes	**Cooking Time:** 0 minutes	**Servings:** 2

INGREDIENTS:

1 cup muesli 2 cups skim milk	Fresh or dried fruit for topping (optional)	Honey or maple syrup for sweetness (optional)

INSTRUCTIONS:

1.Divide the muesli into two bowls.
2.Pour skim milk over the muesli in each bowl.
3.Let it sit for a few minutes to allow the muesli to soften slightly.
4.Top with fresh or dried fruit and a drizzle of honey or maple syrup if desired.

NUTRITIONAL VALUES (PER SERVING):

✓ Calories: Approximately 220 ✓ Protein: 12g	✓ Fat: 2g ✓ Carbohydrates: 40g	✓ Fiber: 4g

PREPARATION TIPS:

- For a creamier texture, you can soak the muesli in milk overnight in the refrigerator.
- Mixing in a spoonful of yogurt can add creaminess and a probiotic boost.

SHOPPING TIPS:

- Look for muesli mixes that contain a variety of grains, nuts, and seeds for maximum nutritional benefits.
- Choosing low-fat or non-fat milk helps keep the breakfast light yet satisfying.

ALTERNATIVE VARIATIONS:

- Use almond milk or another plant-based milk for a dairy-free option.
- Stir in a spoonful of nut butter for added flavor and healthy fats.

18) NUT BUTTER AND JELLY OATMEAL

Preparation Time: 5 minutes	**Cooking Time:** 10 minutes	**Servings:** 2

INGREDIENTS:

1 cup rolled oats 2 cups water or milk	2 tablespoons nut butter (peanut, almond, or cashew) 2 tablespoons jelly or jam of your choice	Fresh berries or sliced bananas (optional, for topping)

INSTRUCTIONS:

1. In a medium saucepan, bring the water or milk to a boil. Add the oats, reducing the heat to simmer, stirring occasionally until the oats are soft and have absorbed the liquid, about 5 minutes.
2. Stir in the nut butter and jelly until evenly distributed throughout the oatmeal.
3. Serve the oatmeal hot, topped with fresh berries or sliced bananas if using.

NUTRITIONAL VALUES (PER SERVING):

✓ Calories: 330 ✓ Protein: 10g	✓ Fat: 14g ✓ Carbohydrates: 44g	✓ Fiber: 6g

PREPARATION TIPS:

- Choose natural, unsweetened nut butter and low-sugar jellies to keep this meal as healthy as possible.
- For creamier oatmeal, opt for milk instead of water.

SHOPPING TIPS:

- For oatmeal, choosing old-fashioned oats offers a better texture and nutritional profile than instant varieties.
- When selecting jelly or jam, opt for brands that use real fruit and have no added sugars or high-fructose corn syrup.

ALTERNATIVE VARIATIONS:

- Swap out the jelly for fresh fruit compote for a less processed sweetener.
- Incorporate a scoop of protein powder or Greek yogurt for an extra protein boost.

19) OATMEAL WITH APPLES AND CINNAMON

Preparation Time: 5 minutes	**Cooking Time:** 10 minutes	**Servings:** 2

INGREDIENTS:

1 cup rolled oats 2 cups water or milk (for creamier oatmeal) 1 apple, cored and diced	1/2 teaspoon cinnamon 1 tablespoon honey or maple syrup (optional) A pinch of salt	Chopped nuts or seeds for topping (optional)

INSTRUCTIONS:

1. In a medium saucepan, bring the water or milk to a boil. Add a pinch of salt.
2. Stir in the rolled oats and diced apple. Reduce heat and simmer for 5 minutes, stirring occasionally.
3. Once the oatmeal has thickened to your liking, remove it from heat. Stir in the cinnamon and sweeten with honey or maple syrup if desired.
4. Serve the oatmeal hot, garnished with additional apple slices, a sprinkle of cinnamon, and chopped nuts or seeds if using.

NUTRITIONAL VALUES (PER SERVING):

✓ Calories: 220 ✓ Protein: 6g	✓ Fat: 3g ✓ Carbohydrates: 45g	✓ Fiber: 6g

PREPARATION TIPS:

- Soaking the oats overnight can reduce cooking time and make the oatmeal even creamier.
- Experiment with different types of apples for varying levels of sweetness and tartness.

SHOPPING TIPS:

- Choose old-fashioned rolled oats for the best texture; avoid instant oats for a less processed option.
- Organic apples and local honey can enhance the flavor and health benefits of your oatmeal.

ALTERNATIVE VARIATIONS:

- Swap out apples for pears or peaches depending on the season.
- Add a spoonful of nut butter for extra creaminess and a boost of protein.

20) Omelet with Mushrooms and Onions

Preparation Time: 10 minutes	**Cooking Time:** 5 minutes	**Servings:** 2

INGREDIENTS:

4 large eggs	2 tablespoons milk	Fresh herbs for garnish (optional)
1/2 cup sliced mushrooms	Salt and pepper to taste	
1/4 cup diced onions	1 tablespoon olive oil	

INSTRUCTIONS:

1. In a bowl, whisk together eggs, milk, salt, and pepper.
2. Heat olive oil in a skillet over medium heat. Add onions and mushrooms, and sauté until softened.
3. Pour the egg mixture over the sautéed vegetables. Cook until the edges start to set, then gently lift, and let the uncooked eggs flow underneath.
4. Fold the omelet in half and cook until the eggs are set but still moist.
5. Serve hot, garnished with fresh herbs if desired.

NUTRITIONAL VALUES (PER SERVING):

✓ Calories: Approximately 250	✓ Fat: 18g	✓ Fiber: 1g
✓ Protein: 14g	✓ Carbohydrates: 6g	

PREPARATION TIPS:

- Ensure not to overcook the omelet to maintain its moistness and flavor.
- Experiment with adding different vegetables or cheese for variety.

SHOPPING TIPS:

- Fresh, organic eggs tend to have a richer flavor and are often more nutritious.
- Select firm, fresh mushrooms and store them properly for the best taste.

ALTERNATIVE VARIATIONS:

- For a dairy-free version, omit the milk or use a plant-based milk alternative.
- Incorporate other vegetables such as spinach, bell peppers, or tomatoes for added nutrients and color.

21) Overnight Oats with Mango

Preparation Time: 8 minutes	**Cooking Time:** 0 minutes	**Servings:** 2

INGREDIENTS:

1 cup rolled oats	2 tablespoons chia seeds	A pinch of cinnamon (optional)
1 cup almond milk (or milk of choice)	1 tablespoon honey or maple syrup (optional)	
1 ripe mango, diced		

INSTRUCTIONS:

1. In a medium bowl, mix the rolled oats and almond milk. Add the chia seeds and a pinch of cinnamon for extra flavor, if desired.
2. Cover and leave the mixture in the refrigerator overnight. The oats and chia seeds will absorb the milk, creating a pudding-like consistency.
3. In the morning, stir the oat mixture. If it's too thick, you can adjust the consistency by adding a bit more milk.
4. Top with diced mango and drizzle with honey or maple syrup for a touch of sweetness if you like.

NUTRITIONAL VALUES (PER SERVING):

✓ Calories: 300	✓ Fat: 5g	✓ Fiber: 9g
✓ Protein: 8g	✓ Carbohydrates: 55g	

PREPARATION TIPS:

- Soaking the oats overnight not only softens them but also makes them easier to digest.
- For an extra creamy texture, you can mix in a tablespoon of Greek yogurt in the morning.

SHOPPING TIPS:

- When choosing mangoes, look for ones that are slightly soft to the touch and have a fruity aroma at their stem ends.

ALTERNATIVE VARIATIONS:

- If mangoes are not in season, you can substitute with frozen mango or another fresh fruit like berries or peaches.
- For a nut-free version, use soy or coconut milk instead of almond milk.

22) Overnight Oats with Peanut Butter

Preparation Time: 10 minutes	**Cooking Time:** 0 minutes	**Servings:** 2

INGREDIENTS:

1 cup rolled oats	1 tablespoon chia seeds	A pinch of cinnamon (optional)
1 1/2 cups almond milk (or any milk of choice)	2 tablespoons honey or maple syrup (adjust to taste)	
2 tablespoons peanut butter	1 ripe banana, sliced	

INSTRUCTIONS:

1. In a bowl, combine rolled oats, almond milk, peanut butter, chia seeds, and honey or maple syrup. Mix well to ensure all the oats are soaked.
2. Cover the bowl and refrigerate overnight, allowing the oats to absorb the liquid and soften.
3. In the morning, stir the oat mixture to check consistency. Add a little more milk if it's too thick.
4. Serve the oats in bowls or jars, topped with sliced banana and a sprinkle of cinnamon if desired.

NUTRITIONAL VALUES (PER SERVING):

| ✓ Calories: 380 | ✓ Fat: 14g | ✓ Fiber: 9g |
| ✓ Protein: 12g | ✓ Carbohydrates: 56g | |

PREPARATION TIPS:

- Warm the peanut butter slightly for easier mixing with the oats and milk.
- For a crunchy texture, top with granola or nuts just before serving.

SHOPPING TIPS:

- Select a high-quality, natural peanut butter with no added sugars or oils for the healthiest option.
- Rolled oats are preferred for their texture; opt for organic if possible.

ALTERNATIVE VARIATIONS:

- Swap peanut butter with almond or cashew butter for a different flavor profile.
- Add cocoa powder to the mixture for a chocolatey twist.

23) PROTEIN PANCAKES

Preparation Time: 10 minutes	**Cooking Time:** 5 minutes	**Servings:** 2

INGREDIENTS:

1 cup oat flour (or whole wheat flour)	1/2 teaspoon cinnamon	1 tablespoon maple syrup (plus more for serving)
2 scoops vanilla protein powder	2 egg whites	
1/2 teaspoon baking powder	1 cup almond milk	1/2 cup mixed berries (for topping)

INSTRUCTIONS:

1. In a large bowl, mix oat flour, protein powder, baking powder, and cinnamon.
2. In another bowl, whisk together egg whites, almond milk, and maple syrup until well combined.
3. Pour the wet ingredients into the dry ingredients and stir until just combined. Let the batter sit for 5 minutes to thicken slightly.
4. Heat a non-stick skillet over medium heat and lightly grease it with cooking spray or oil. Pour 1/4 cup of batter onto the skillet for each pancake. Cook until bubbles form on the surface, then flip and cook until golden brown on the other side.
5. Serve the pancakes topped with fresh berries and a drizzle of maple syrup.

NUTRITIONAL VALUES (PER SERVING):

| ✓ Calories: 350 | ✓ Fat: 5g | ✓ Fiber: 6g |
| ✓ Protein: 25g | ✓ Carbohydrates: 50g | |

PREPARATION TIPS:

- Allow the batter to rest before cooking to ensure fluffy pancakes.
- For an extra protein boost, add a tablespoon of Greek yogurt to the batter.

SHOPPING TIPS:

- Look for a protein powder that's low in sugar and high in protein content.
- Fresh, in-season berries will provide the best flavor and nutritional value.

ALTERNATIVE VARIATIONS:

- Substitute almond milk with any other milk of your choice.
- Try adding different fruits or nuts into the batter for variety.

24) SCRAMBLED EGGS WITH SPINACH AND FETA

Preparation Time: 5 minutes	**Cooking Time:** 5 minutes	**Servings:** 2

INGREDIENTS:

| 4 large eggs | 1/4 cup feta cheese, crumbled | 1 tablespoon olive oil |
| 1 cup fresh spinach, chopped | Salt and pepper to taste | |

INSTRUCTIONS:

1. Beat the eggs in a bowl and season with salt and pepper.
2. Heat the olive oil in a non-stick pan over medium heat. Add the spinach and sauté until just wilted, about 1-2 minutes.
3. Pour the beaten eggs over the spinach in the pan. Let them sit, undisturbed, for a few seconds, then gently stir them with a spatula.
4. When the eggs are almost set but still slightly runny, sprinkle the crumbled feta cheese over the top. Continue cooking until the cheese is slightly melted and the eggs are cooked to your liking.
5. Serve the scrambled eggs warm, with additional salt and pepper if needed.

NUTRITIONAL VALUES (PER SERVING):

| ✓ Calories: 250 | ✓ Fat: 18g | ✓ Fiber: 1g |
| ✓ Protein: 18g | ✓ Carbohydrates: 2g | |

- For a fluffier texture, add a splash of milk to the eggs before beating them.
- Adjust the cooking time if you prefer your scrambled eggs firm.

SHOPPING TIPS:

- Choose fresh, organic spinach for the best flavor and nutritional value.
- Look for feta cheese that is stored in brine for added moisture and flavor.

ALTERNATIVE VARIATIONS:

- Add cherry tomatoes or mushrooms for an extra serving of vegetables.
- Swap feta cheese with goat cheese for a different creamy element.

25) SCRAMBLED TOFU WITH SPINACH AND TOMATOES

Preparation Time: 10 minutes	**Cooking Time:** 8 minutes	**Servings:** 2

INGREDIENTS:

1 block (14 oz) firm tofu, drained and crumbled 1 tablespoon olive oil	1 cup fresh spinach, chopped 1/2 cup cherry tomatoes, halved 1/4 teaspoon turmeric (for color)	Salt and pepper to taste Nutritional yeast (optional, for a cheesy flavor)

INSTRUCTIONS:

1. Heat the olive oil in a skillet over medium heat. Add the crumbled tofu and turmeric and cook for 2-3 minutes until the tofu starts to get some color.
2. Stir in the spinach and cook until just wilted about 2 minutes.
3. Add the cherry tomatoes and cook for another 2-3 minutes, until they're just soft.
4. Season with salt, pepper, and nutritional yeast if using. Serve warm.

NUTRITIONAL VALUES (PER SERVING):

✓ Calories: Approximately 250 ✓ Protein: 18g	✓ Fat: 15g ✓ Carbohydrates: 8g	✓ Fiber: 3g

PREPARATION TIPS:

- Press the tofu before cooking to remove excess water and achieve a better texture.
- Add a dash of black salt (kala namak) for an eggy flavor.

SHOPPING TIPS:

- Choose organic tofu and fresh, local produce, when possible, for the best taste and nutritional value.

ALTERNATIVE VARIATIONS:

- Incorporate different vegetables, such as bell peppers or onions, for more variety and color.
- Spice it up with a sprinkle of chili flakes or hot sauce for an extra kick.

26) SMOOTHIE BOWL WITH NUTS AND SEEDS

Preparation Time: 10 minutes	**Cooking Time:** 0 minutes	**Servings:** 2

INGREDIENTS:

1 frozen banana 1/2 cup mixed berries (fresh or frozen) 1/2 cup almond milk (or any milk of choice)	1 tablespoon chia seeds 1 tablespoon flaxseed 1/4 cup mixed nuts (almonds, walnuts, cashews), chopped	A sprinkle of coconut flakes A few berries and mint leaves for garnish

INSTRUCTIONS:

1. In a blender, combine the frozen banana, mixed berries, and almond milk. Blend until smooth.
2. Pour the smoothie mixture into two bowls.
3. Top each bowl with chia seeds, flaxseed, chopped nuts, and coconut flakes evenly.
4. Garnish with a few additional berries and mint leaves for a refreshing touch.

NUTRITIONAL VALUES (PER SERVING):

✓ Calories: 300 ✓ Protein: 8g	✓ Fat: 15g ✓ Carbohydrates: 35g	✓ Fiber: 9g

PREPARATION TIPS:

- For a thicker smoothie bowl, use less milk or add a scoop of your favorite protein powder.
- Freeze your fruits ahead of time for a cold, creamy texture.

SHOPPING TIPS:

- Opt for unsweetened almond milk to keep the sugar content low.
- Choose ripe bananas for natural sweetness and creamy texture.

ALTERNATIVE VARIATIONS:

- Mix up the fruits based on seasonality and personal preference.
- For added sweetness, drizzle with honey or maple syrup.

27) SPINACH AND BANANA SMOOTHIE

Preparation Time: 5 minutes	**Cooking Time:** 0 minutes	**Servings:** 2

INGREDIENTS:

2 ripe bananas 2 cups fresh spinach leaves 1 cup Greek yogurt (for added protein)	1 cup almond milk (or water for a lighter version)	Ice cubes (optional, for a colder smoothie)

INSTRUCTIONS:

1. Place bananas, spinach, Greek yogurt, and almond milk in a blender. Add ice cubes if desired.
2. Blend until smooth and creamy. Adjust the consistency by adding more almond milk or water if necessary.
3. Taste and add a bit of honey or maple syrup if you prefer a sweeter smoothie.
4. Serve immediately, enjoying the energy boost and nutrient-rich start to your day.

NUTRITIONAL VALUES (PER SERVING):

✓ Calories: 210 ✓ Protein: 12g	✓ Fat: 3g ✓ Carbohydrates: 37g	✓ Fiber: 5g

PREPARATION TIPS:

- Freeze the bananas ahead of time for a thicker, creamier smoothie.
- Add a tablespoon of chia seeds or flaxseed for an omega-3 boost.

SHOPPING TIPS:

- Choose ripe bananas for natural sweetness; frozen bananas work great for a thicker smoothie.
- Fresh spinach should be vibrant and green without any signs of wilting.
- Organic spinach is recommended to minimize pesticide exposure.

ALTERNATIVE VARIATIONS:

- Include a scoop of your favorite protein powder for an extra protein kick.
- Mix in other fruits like mango or pineapple for added sweetness and tropical flavors.

28) SPINACH AND FETA OMELET

Preparation Time: 5 minutes	**Cooking Time:** 5 minutes	**Servings:** 2

INGREDIENTS:

4 large eggs 1 cup fresh spinach, chopped	1/4 cup feta cheese, crumbled 2 tablespoons milk	Salt and pepper to taste 1 tablespoon olive oil

INSTRUCTIONS:

1. In a bowl, whisk together eggs, milk, salt, and pepper until well combined.
2. Heat olive oil in a non-stick skillet over medium heat.
3. Add spinach to the skillet and sauté until just wilted, about 1-2 minutes.
4. Pour the egg mixture over the spinach. Cook for a few minutes until the edges start to set.
5. Sprinkle feta cheese over half of the omelet. Fold the other half over the cheese and continue cooking until the cheese is melted and the eggs are set to your liking.
6. Carefully slide the omelet onto a plate and serve warm.

NUTRITIONAL VALUES (PER SERVING):

✓ Calories: 250 ✓ Protein: 18g	✓ Fat: 18g ✓ Carbohydrates: 2g	✓ Fiber: 0.5g

PREPARATION TIPS:

- Whisking the eggs thoroughly before cooking ensures a fluffy omelet.
- Feel free to add other vegetables like tomatoes or bell peppers for extra flavor and nutrients.

SHOPPING TIPS:

- Select fresh, bright green spinach leaves for the best taste and nutritional value.
- Look for high-quality, creamy feta cheese for the best flavor in your omelet.

ALTERNATIVE VARIATIONS:

- Substitute spinach with kale or arugula for a different green option.
- Add mushrooms or onions for an extra layer of flavor.

29) BREAKFAST: SPINACH AND FETA BREAKFAST WRAP

Preparation Time: 10 minutes	**Cooking Time:** 5 minutes	**Servings:** 2

INGREDIENTS:

2 whole-grain tortillas 4 eggs, beaten 1 cup fresh spinach, chopped	1/2 cup feta cheese, crumbled 1 tablespoon olive oil Salt and pepper to taste	*Optional:* cherry tomatoes, sliced for added freshness

INSTRUCTIONS:

1.Heat olive oil in a non-stick skillet over medium heat. Add the beaten eggs and scramble until they are just set.
2.Stir in the chopped spinach and cook until the spinach has wilted. Season with salt and pepper.
3.Warm the tortillas in the microwave for about 10-15 seconds to make them more pliable.
4.Divide the scrambled eggs and spinach mixture evenly among the tortillas. Sprinkle crumbled feta cheese over the top.
5.If using, add a few slices of cherry tomatoes onto each wrap for a burst of flavor and color.
6.Fold the sides of the tortilla in, then roll it up tightly. Serve immediately.

NUTRITIONAL INFORMATION (PER SERVING):

| ✓ Calories: 320 | ✓ Fat: 20g | ✓ Fiber: 3g |
| ✓ Protein: 20g | ✓ Carbohydrates: 20g | |

PREPARATION TIPS:

For an extra fluffy scramble, add a splash of milk to the eggs before beating.

SHOPPING TIPS:

- Opt for high-quality, whole-grain tortillas for added fiber and nutrients. Fresh, organic spinach and free-range eggs will enhance the flavor and health benefits of your wrap.

ALTERNATIVE VARIATIONS:

- For a twist, add sautéed mushrooms or onions to the filling, or use kale instead of spinach for a different green option. To keep it low carb, you can skip the tortilla and enjoy it as a hearty scramble.

30) WHOLE GRAIN TOAST WITH ALMOND BUTTER

| **Preparation Time:** 5 minutes | **Cooking Time:** 2 minutes | **Servings:** 2 |

INGREDIENTS:

| 2 slices of whole-grain bread
2 tablespoons almond butter | 1 banana, sliced (or strawberries, depending on preference) | A sprinkle of chia seeds (optional)
Honey (optional) |

INSTRUCTIONS:

1.Toast the whole-grain bread slices to your desired level of crispiness.
2.Spread a tablespoon of almond butter on each slice of toast.
3.Arrange the banana slices (or strawberry slices) on top of the almond butter.
4.For an added boost of nutrition and texture, sprinkle chia seeds over the top.
5.Drizzle with honey for a touch of sweetness, if desired.

NUTRITIONAL VALUES (PER SERVING):

| ✓ Calories: 280 | ✓ Fat: 14g | ✓ Fiber: 6g |
| ✓ Protein: 8g | ✓ Carbohydrates: 32g | |

PREPARATION TIPS:

- Experiment with different types of whole-grain bread to find your favorite.
- Warming the almond butter slightly can make it easier to spread.

SHOPPING TIPS:

- Look for bread that has "whole grain" as the first ingredient and contains minimal added sugars.
- Opt for natural almond butter without added sugars or palm oil.

ALTERNATIVE VARIATIONS:

- Substitute almond butter with peanut butter or cashew butter for a different flavor.
- Add a layer of fresh spinach or arugula for a savory twist.

31) WHOLE WHEAT PANCAKES WITH BLUEBERRIES

| **Preparation Time:** 15 minutes | **Cooking Time:** 10 minutes | **Servings:** 2 |

INGREDIENTS:

| 1 cup whole wheat flour
2 teaspoons baking powder
1/2 teaspoon salt
1 tablespoon sugar (optional) | 1 cup milk (any kind)
1 egg
2 tablespoons unsalted butter, melted, plus more for cooking | 1/2 cup fresh blueberries (plus more for serving)
Maple syrup, for serving |

INSTRUCTIONS:

1.In a large bowl, whisk together the whole wheat flour, baking powder, salt, and sugar (if using).
2.In another bowl, beat the milk, egg, and melted butter until well combined.
3.Pour the wet ingredients into the dry ingredients, stirring until just combined (it's okay if the batter is a little lumpy). Gently fold in the blueberries.
4.Heat a non-stick skillet or griddle over medium heat and brush with a little butter. Pour 1/4 cup of batter for each pancake and cook until bubbles appear on the surface and the edges look set, about 2-3 minutes. Flip and cook for another 2 minutes or until golden brown.
5.Serve the pancakes warm, topped with additional blueberries and maple syrup.

NUTRITIONAL VALUES (PER SERVING):

| ✓ Calories: Approximately 350 | ✓ Protein: 10g | ✓ Fat: 12g |

✓ Carbohydrates: 52g | ✓ Fiber: 8g

PREPARATION TIPS:

- Don't overmix the batter; lumps are perfectly fine and will help keep the pancakes light and fluffy.
- For an added nutritional boost, mix a tablespoon of ground flaxseed or chia seeds into the batter.

SHOPPING TIPS:

- When buying whole wheat flour, look for 100% whole grain to ensure you're getting the full benefits of the wheat kernel.
- Choose high-quality, pure maple syrup for the best flavor and health benefits.

ALTERNATIVE VARIATIONS:

- Substitute blueberries with other berries like raspberries or sliced strawberries for different flavors.
- For a vegan version, use plant-based milk and a flax egg (1 tablespoon ground flaxseed mixed with 3 tablespoons water).

32) *YOGURT WITH GRANOLA AND HONEY*

Preparation Time: 5 minutes	**Cooking Time:** 0 minutes	**Servings:** 2

INGREDIENTS:

2 cups plain or vanilla Greek yogurt 1/2 cup granola	2 tablespoons honey	Fresh fruit for topping (optional, such as berries or sliced banana)

INSTRUCTIONS:

1. Spoon the Greek yogurt into two bowls.
2. Sprinkle granola over the yogurt in each bowl.
3. Drizzle honey on top of the granola and yogurt.
4. If desired, add fresh fruit on top for additional sweetness and a burst of flavor.

NUTRITIONAL VALUES (PER SERVING):

✓ Calories: Approximately 300 ✓ Protein: 20g	✓ Fat: 7g ✓ Carbohydrates: 42g	✓ Fiber: 2g

PREPARATION TIPS:

- For a lower-sugar option, choose plain Greek yogurt and sweeten it yourself with a bit of honey or maple syrup.
- To keep the granola crunchy, add it just before serving.

SHOPPING TIPS:

- Look for granola with a short ingredient list to avoid unnecessary sugars and additives.
- Buying bulk Greek yogurt can be more cost-effective and environmentally friendly.

ALTERNATIVE VARIATIONS:

- Mix in a scoop of your favorite protein powder with the yogurt for an extra protein boost.
- For a dairy-free version, substitute Greek yogurt with a plant-based alternative like almond or coconut yogurt.

33) ASIAN CHICKEN SALAD

Preparation Time: 20 minutes	**Cooking Time:** 10 minutes (if cooking chicken)	**Servings:** 2

INGREDIENTS:

2 cups cooked chicken, shredded	1/4 cup sliced almonds	1 teaspoon honey
2 cups mixed salad greens	For the dressing:	1 garlic clove, minced
1/2 cup shredded carrots	2 tablespoons soy sauce	1 teaspoon grated fresh ginger
1/2 cup sliced red cabbage	1 tablespoon sesame oil	
1/4 cup chopped green onions	1 tablespoon rice vinegar	

INSTRUCTIONS:

1. In a large bowl, combine the salad greens, shredded carrots, red cabbage, green onions, and shredded chicken.
2. In a small bowl, whisk together all the ingredients for the dressing until well combined.
3. Pour the dressing over the salad and toss until everything is evenly coated.
4. Sprinkle sliced almonds on top before serving.

NUTRITIONAL VALUES (PER SERVING):

✓ Calories: Approximately 320	✓ Fat: 18g	✓ Fiber: 3g
✓ Protein: 30g	✓ Carbohydrates: 12g	

PREPARATION TIPS:

- Cooking the chicken in advance or using leftover chicken can save time when preparing this salad.
- Let the salad sit for a few minutes after adding the dressing to allow the flavors to meld.

SHOPPING TIPS:

- Look for pre-cooked, rotisserie chicken for convenience, ensuring it's not heavily seasoned.
- Fresh ingredients are key for the salad; select vibrant vegetables for the best taste and nutritional value.

ALTERNATIVE VARIATIONS:

- Swap chicken for tofu or tempeh for a vegetarian version.
- Add mandarin orange slices or sesame seeds for extra flavor and texture.

34) ASIAN NOODLE SALAD

Preparation Time: 20 minutes	**Cooking Time:** 0 minutes (assuming noodles are pre-cooked)	**Servings:** 2

INGREDIENTS:

2 cups cooked noodles (soba, rice noodles, or spaghetti work well)	1/2 cucumber, julienned	1 tablespoon sesame oil
1 cup shredded cabbage	1/4 cup chopped green onions	1 tablespoon rice vinegar
1 carrot, julienned	1/4 cup chopped cilantro	1 teaspoon honey or sugar
1 bell pepper, thinly sliced	***For the dressing:***	1 garlic clove, minced
	2 tablespoons soy sauce	1 teaspoon grated ginger

INSTRUCTIONS:

1. In a large bowl, combine the cooked noodles with the cabbage, carrot, bell pepper, cucumber, green onions, and cilantro.
2. In a small bowl, whisk together the ingredients for the dressing until well combined.
3. Pour the dressing over the noodle mixture and toss to evenly coat all the ingredients.
4. Chill the salad in the refrigerator for at least 30 minutes before serving to allow the flavors to meld.

NUTRITIONAL VALUES (PER SERVING):

✓ Calories: Approximately 350	✓ Fat: 9g	✓ Fiber: 4g
✓ Protein: 8g	✓ Carbohydrates: 60g	

PREPARATION TIPS:

- Chilling the salad before serving enhances the flavors and provides a refreshing taste.
- Toasted sesame seeds or chopped peanuts can be sprinkled on top for added crunch.

SHOPPING TIPS:

- For the freshest vegetables, select those that are firm and vibrant in color.
- Various types of noodles are available in the international or Asian section of most supermarkets.

ALTERNATIVE VARIATIONS:

- Add grilled chicken, shrimp, or tofu for additional protein.
- For a spicier salad, include a dash of chili sauce or chili flakes in the dressing.

35) AVOCADO CHICKEN SALAD

Preparation Time: 15 minutes	Cooking Time: 0 minutes (assuming pre-cooked chicken)	Servings: 2

INGREDIENTS:

2 cups cooked chicken, shredded, or diced 1 ripe avocado, diced 1/2 cucumber, diced	1/2 red bell pepper, diced 1/4 red onion, thinly sliced Juice of 1 lime 2 tablespoons olive oil	Salt and pepper to taste Fresh cilantro, chopped (optional, for garnish)

INSTRUCTIONS:

1. In a large bowl, combine the chicken, avocado, cucumber, bell pepper, and red onion.
2. In a small bowl, whisk together lime juice, olive oil, salt, and pepper to create the dressing.
3. Pour the dressing over the salad and gently toss to combine, ensuring not to mash the avocado.
4. Adjust seasoning as needed.
5. Serve the salad chilled or at room temperature, garnished with cilantro if desired.

NUTRITIONAL VALUES (PER SERVING):

✓ Calories: 450 ✓ Protein: 35g	✓ Fat: 30g ✓ Carbohydrates: 12g	✓ Fiber: 7g

PREPARATION TIPS:

- Chill the cooked chicken and avocado before assembling the salad to keep it fresh and cool.
- Lemon juice can be substituted for lime juice for a different citrus twist.

SHOPPING TIPS:

- Opt for a rotisserie chicken for convenience or cook and shred your chicken breast to control the seasoning.
- Avocados should be ripe but firm to ensure they mix well without becoming mushy in the salad.

ALTERNATIVE VARIATIONS:

- Swap chicken for canned tuna or chickpeas for a different protein source.
- Include cherry tomatoes or corn for additional sweetness and color.

36) BEET AND GOAT CHEESE ARUGULA SALAD

Preparation Time: 15 minutes (plus beet roasting time)	Cooking Time: 45-60 minutes for roasting beets	Servings: 2

INGREDIENTS:

2 medium beets, roasted, peeled, and sliced 4 cups arugula	1/2 cup goat cheese, crumbled 1/4 cup walnuts, toasted and chopped 2 tablespoons balsamic vinaigrette	Salt and pepper to taste Optional garnishes: orange segments, fresh herbs

INSTRUCTIONS:

1. To roast the beets, wrap them individually in foil and bake at 400°F (200°C) until tender, about 45-60 minutes. Once cool enough to handle, peel and slice.
2. In a large bowl, toss the arugula with the balsamic vinaigrette until lightly coated.
3. Arrange the dressed arugula on plates, then top with sliced beets, crumbled goat cheese, and toasted walnuts.
4. Season with salt and pepper to taste. Add optional garnishes like orange segments or fresh herbs for additional flavor and color.

NUTRITIONAL VALUES (PER SERVING):

✓ Calories: Approximately 300 ✓ Protein: 10g	✓ Fat: 20g ✓ Carbohydrates: 20g	✓ Fiber: 5g

PREPARATION TIPS:

- Roasting beets ahead of time and storing them in the refrigerator can save on preparation time.
- To easily peel the roasted beets, use a paper towel to rub the skin off once they are cool.

SHOPPING TIPS:

- Select firm, smooth beets without any visible damage or soft spots.
- Fresh, young arugula leaves tend to be less bitter and more tender.

ALTERNATIVE VARIATIONS:

- Substitute walnuts with pecans or almonds for a different crunch.
- For a dairy-free version, replace goat cheese with avocado slices or a dairy-free cheese alternative.

37) BROCCOLI CHEDDAR SOUP

Preparation Time: 10 minutes	Cooking Time: 30 minutes	Servings: 2

INGREDIENTS:

2 cups broccoli florets	1 garlic clove, minced	1 cup milk
1 tablespoon butter	2 tablespoons flour	1 cup shredded sharp cheddar cheese
1 small onion, diced	2 cups vegetable broth	Salt and pepper to taste

INSTRUCTIONS:

1. In a large pot, melt the butter over medium heat. Add the diced onion and garlic, sautéing until soft and translucent.
2. Sprinkle the flour over the onions and garlic, stirring to form a roux. Cook for a couple of minutes.
3. Gradually add the vegetable broth, whisking constantly to avoid lumps. Bring to a simmer.
4. Add the broccoli florets to the pot. Cover and simmer until the broccoli are tender, about 15-20 minutes.
5. Stir in the milk and shredded cheese, continuing to cook until the cheese is melted, and the soup is heated through. Season with salt and pepper.
6. Use an immersion blender to partially blend the soup for a creamy yet chunky texture.

NUTRITIONAL VALUES (PER SERVING):

| ✓ Calories: Approximately 400 | ✓ Fat: 25g | ✓ Fiber: 3g |
| ✓ Protein: 20g | ✓ Carbohydrates: 25g | |

PREPARATION TIPS:

- For a smoother soup, blend all the soup until creamy. Adjust the thickness by adding more milk or broth if necessary.
- Reserve some broccoli florets to add after blending for added texture.

SHOPPING TIPS:

- Choose fresh, bright green broccoli with firm florets.
- For the best flavor, opt for sharp or extra-sharp cheddar cheese.

ALTERNATIVE VARIATIONS:

- Substitute broccoli with cauliflower for a different take on the soup.
- For a lighter version, use low-fat milk and reduced-fat cheese.

38) CAPRESE PASTA SALAD

| **Preparation Time:** 15 minutes | **Cooking Time:** 10 minutes | **Servings:** 2 |

INGREDIENTS:

2 cups cooked pasta (such as farfalle, penne, or fusilli)	8 oz fresh mozzarella cheese, cubed or use mini mozzarella balls	2 tablespoons extra virgin olive oil
1 cup cherry tomatoes, halved	1/4 cup fresh basil leaves, torn	1 tablespoon balsamic glaze
		Salt and pepper to taste

INSTRUCTIONS:

1. In a large bowl, combine the cooked pasta, cherry tomatoes, and mozzarella cheese.
2. Add the fresh basil leaves to the pasta mixture.
3. Drizzle the olive oil and balsamic glaze over the salad. Gently toss to ensure all ingredients are evenly coated.
4. Season with salt and pepper to taste.
5. Serve the salad at room temperature or chilled, as preferred.

NUTRITIONAL VALUES (PER SERVING):

| • Calories: Approximately 450 | • Fat: 20g | • Fiber: 3g |
| • Protein: 22g | • Carbohydrates: 48g | |

PREPARATION TIPS:

- For the best flavor, allow the pasta salad to marinate for at least 30 minutes in the refrigerator before serving.
- Cooking the pasta al dente ensures it retains a nice texture when mixed with the other ingredients.

SHOPPING TIPS:

- Choose high-quality fresh mozzarella for its creamy texture and mild flavor.
- Look for ripe but firm cherry tomatoes for the best taste and texture in your salad.

ALTERNATIVE VARIATIONS:

- Add grilled chicken or shrimp to turn this salad into a more substantial meal.
- For a vegan version, substitute the mozzarella with vegan cheese or avocado for creaminess.

39) CHICKPEA VEGGIE WRAPS

| **Preparation Time:** 15 minutes | **Cooking Time:** 0 minutes | **Servings:** 2 |

INGREDIENTS:

1 can (15 oz) chickpeas, drained and rinsed	1 carrot, grated	1 handful of baby spinach leaves
2 whole wheat tortillas	1/2 cucumber, thinly sliced	Salt and pepper to taste
1 avocado, sliced	1/2 bell pepper, thinly sliced	
	2 tablespoons hummus	

INSTRUCTIONS:

1. In a bowl, lightly mash the chickpeas with a fork. Mix in salt and pepper to taste.
2. Spread hummus on each tortilla, then add an even layer of mashed chickpeas.

3.Top with avocado slices, grated carrot, cucumber slices, bell pepper slices, and baby spinach.

4.Roll up the tortillas tightly, folding them in the sides to enclose the filling.

5.Cut each wrap in half and serve immediately.

NUTRITIONAL VALUES (PER SERVING):

✓ Calories: Approximately 350	✓ Fat: 15g	✓ Fiber: 10g
✓ Protein: 12g	✓ Carbohydrates: 45g	

PREPARATION TIPS:

- For added flavor, consider incorporating a sprinkle of paprika or cumin into the chickpea mixture.
- Warming the tortillas slightly will make them more pliable and easier to wrap.

SHOPPING TIPS:

- Choose ripe avocados for their creaminess. Test for ripeness by gently pressing the skin; it should yield slightly under pressure.
- When selecting tortillas, opt for whole wheat for a healthier option that provides extra fiber.

ALTERNATIVE VARIATIONS:

- Swap hummus for tzatziki sauce for a different flavor profile.
- Add roasted red peppers or sun-dried tomatoes for an additional sweet and tangy taste.

40) CLASSIC CAESAR SALAD WITH GRILLED CHICKEN

Preparation Time: 15 minutes	**Cooking Time:** 10 minutes	**Servings:** 2

INGREDIENTS:

2 chicken breasts, grilled and sliced 4 cups romaine lettuce, chopped 1/2 cup croutons	1/4 cup Parmesan cheese, shaved Caesar dressing (store-bought or homemade)	Salt and pepper to taste Lemon wedges, for serving

INSTRUCTIONS:

1.In a large bowl, combine the chopped romaine lettuce with enough Caesar dressing to coat the leaves lightly. Toss well.

2.Divide the dressed lettuce between two plates. Top each salad with sliced grilled chicken, croutons, and shaved Parmesan cheese.

3.Season with salt and pepper to taste.

4.Serve with lemon wedges on the side for an extra burst of freshness.

NUTRITIONAL VALUES (PER SERVING):

✓ Calories: Approximately 400	✓ Fat: 20g	✓ Fiber: 2g
✓ Protein: 35g	✓ Carbohydrates: 15g	

PREPARATION TIPS:

- Grilling the chicken adds a smoky flavor that complements the creamy dressing and crisp lettuce.
- Homemade Caesar dressing can be made healthier with Greek yogurt as a base.

SHOPPING TIPS:

- Opt for fresh, crisp romaine lettuce for the best texture in your salad.
- When buying Parmesan cheese, choose a block and shave it yourself for the freshest flavor.

ALTERNATIVE VARIATIONS:

- For a vegetarian version, omit the chicken and add chickpeas or boiled eggs for protein.
- Include anchovies or bacon bits for traditional Caesar salad lovers seeking extra umami flavors.

41) CURRY CHICKEN SALAD

Preparation Time: 20 minutes	**Cooking Time:** 0 minutes (assuming chicken is pre-cooked)	**Servings:** 2

INGREDIENTS:

2 cups cooked and shredded chicken breast 1/2 cup red grapes, halved	1/4 cup celery, diced 1/4 cup mayonnaise 1 tablespoon curry powder	Salt and pepper to taste Lettuce leaves, for serving

INSTRUCTIONS:

1.In a large bowl, combine the shredded chicken, grapes, and celery.

2.In a small bowl, mix the mayonnaise with the curry powder, salt, and pepper until well blended.

3.Add the curry mayonnaise to the chicken mixture and stir until evenly coated.

4.Chill the salad for at least 30 minutes before serving to enhance the flavors.

5.Serve on a bed of lettuce leaves.

NUTRITIONAL VALUES (PER SERVING):

✓ Calories: Approximately 370	✓ Fat: 20g	✓ Fiber: 2g
✓ Protein: 35g	✓ Carbohydrates: 12g	

PREPARATION TIPS:

- To lighten the dish, you can substitute Greek yogurt for part or all the mayonnaise.
- For extra crunch and nuttiness, add slivered almonds to the salad.

- When buying chicken, opt for breast meat for a leaner option; you can cook it in advance to save time.
- Look for fresh, crisp celery and firm, sweet grapes for the best texture and flavor in your salad.

ALTERNATIVE VARIATIONS:

- Make it vegetarian by using chickpeas instead of chicken.
- Add a diced apple for an extra element of sweetness and crunch.

42) FALAFEL WRAP WITH TZATZIKI SAUCE

Preparation Time: 20 minutes	Cooking Time: 10 minutes	Servings: 2

INGREDIENTS:

4 large falafel balls (store-bought or homemade), halved	1 cup lettuce, shredded	1/4 red onion, thinly sliced
2 large whole wheat pita breads	1 tomato, sliced	1/2 cup tzatziki sauce
	1/4 cucumber, sliced	

INSTRUCTIONS:

1. Warm the pita bread in the oven or on a skillet until soft and pliable.
2. Spread a generous layer of tzatziki sauce over each pita bread.
3. Arrange the falafel halves across the center of each pita.
4. Top with lettuce, tomato slices, cucumber slices, and red onion.
5. Roll up the pita bread around the fillings, tucking in the edges to hold everything in place.
6. Serve immediately, with extra tzatziki sauce on the side if desired.

NUTRITIONAL VALUES (PER SERVING):

✓ Calories: Approximately 500	✓ Fat: 22g	✓ Fiber: 8g
✓ Protein: 18g	✓ Carbohydrates: 60g	

PREPARATION TIPS:

- For a lighter version, use lettuce wraps instead of pita bread.
- To make your falafel, blend chickpeas, herbs, spices, and a little flour, then form into balls and bake or fry.

SHOPPING TIPS:

- When buying pita bread, opt for whole wheat versions for added fiber.
- Look for fresh tzatziki sauce in the refrigerated section of the grocery store, or make your own with Greek yogurt, cucumber, garlic, and dill.

ALTERNATIVE VARIATIONS:

- Add pickled vegetables or olives for an extra tangy flavor.
- For vegan tzatziki, use a plant-based yogurt alternative.

43) GREEK PASTA SALAD

Preparation Time: 15 minutes	Cooking Time: 10 minutes	Servings: 2

INGREDIENTS:

2 cups cooked pasta (penne, fusilli, or rotini work well)	1/4 cup Kalamata olives, pitted and halved	1 teaspoon dried oregano
1/2 cup cherry tomatoes, halved	1/2 cup feta cheese, crumbled	Salt and pepper to taste
1/2 cucumber, diced	2 tablespoons extra virgin olive oil	Fresh parsley, chopped, for garnish
1/4 cup red onion, thinly sliced	Juice of 1 lemon	

INSTRUCTIONS:

1. In a large bowl, combine the cooked pasta, cherry tomatoes, cucumber, red onion, Kalamata olives, and feta cheese.
2. In a small bowl, whisk together the olive oil, lemon juice, dried oregano, salt, and pepper to make the dressing.
3. Pour the dressing over the pasta salad and toss until everything is evenly coated.
4. Garnish with chopped parsley before serving. Serve chilled or at room temperature.

NUTRITIONAL VALUES (PER SERVING):

✓ Calories: Approximately 400	✓ Fat: 18g	✓ Fiber: 3g
✓ Protein: 12g	✓ Carbohydrates: 50g	

PREPARATION TIPS:

- Cooking the pasta until just al dente will ensure it maintains a good texture in the salad.
- Let the salad chill in the refrigerator for an hour before serving to allow the flavors to meld.

SHOPPING TIPS:

- Opt for whole wheat pasta for a healthier option that adds extra fiber to your meal.
- When selecting feta cheese, consider buying it in block form and crumbling it yourself for fresher flavor and better texture.

ALTERNATIVE VARIATIONS:

- Add grilled chicken or chickpeas to increase the protein content of the salad.

- For a gluten-free version, use gluten-free pasta or substitute pasta with quinoa.

44) GRILLED CHEESE WITH TOMATO AND BASIL

Preparation Time: 5 minutes	**Cooking Time:** 10 minutes	**Servings:** 2

INGREDIENTS:

4 slices of sourdough bread 4 slices of cheese (mix of cheddar and mozzarella recommended)	1 tomato, sliced Fresh basil leaves Butter, for grilling	Salt and pepper to taste

INSTRUCTIONS:

1. Butter one side of each bread slice. On the unbuttered side, layer a slice of cheese, tomato slices, a sprinkle of salt and pepper, a few basil leaves, and another slice of cheese. Top with another slice of bread, buttered side up.
2. Heat a skillet over medium heat. Place the sandwiches in the skillet, cooking until the bread is golden brown and the cheese has melted, about 4-5 minutes per side.
3. Serve hot, cutting each sandwich in half if desired.

NUTRITIONAL VALUES (PER SERVING):

✓ Calories: Approximately 500 ✓ Protein: 22g	✓ Fat: 25g ✓ Carbohydrates: 50g	✓ Fiber: 3g

PREPARATION TIPS:

- Experiment with different types of cheese for various flavors and melting qualities.
- Adding a thin spread of pesto on the inside of the bread can introduce an additional layer of flavor.

SHOPPING TIPS:

- Choose high-quality, fresh sourdough bread for the best texture and taste.
- For the tomatoes, look for ripe but firm options to ensure they add moisture without making the sandwich soggy.

ALTERNATIVE VARIATIONS:

- For a meatier version, add cooked bacon or ham to the sandwich.
- Vegan options can be made using plant-based cheese and butter substitutes.

45) GRILLED VEGETABLE AND HUMMUS SANDWICH

Preparation Time: 15 minutes	**Cooking Time:** 10 minutes	**Servings:** 2

INGREDIENTS:

1 zucchini, sliced lengthwise 1 bell pepper, sliced into wide strips 1 small eggplant, sliced into rounds	4 slices whole grain bread 1/4 cup hummus Olive oil for grilling	Salt and pepper to taste

INSTRUCTIONS:

1. Preheat a grill pan over medium heat. Brush the sliced vegetables with olive oil and season with salt and pepper.
2. Grill the vegetables in batches until they are tender and have grill marks, about 3-4 minutes per side.
3. Spread hummus on one side of each bread slice.
4. Assemble the sandwiches by layering the grilled vegetables between two slices of hummus-spread bread.
5. Serve immediately or press in a panini press for a warm sandwich.

NUTRITIONAL VALUES (PER SERVING):

✓ Calories: Approximately 350 ✓ Protein: 12g	✓ Fat: 14g ✓ Carbohydrates: 46g	✓ Fiber: 11g

PREPARATION TIPS:

- For a smokier flavor, grill the vegetables on an outdoor grill.
- Additional toppings like fresh spinach, sliced avocado, or a sprinkle of goat cheese can enhance the sandwich.

SHOPPING TIPS:

- Choose fresh, firm vegetables for grilling. The fresher the produce, the better the flavor and nutritional content.
- Opt for high-quality hummus without unnecessary additives for the healthiest option.

ALTERNATIVE VARIATIONS:

- For a gluten-free version, use gluten-free bread or wrap the grilled vegetables and hummus in large lettuce leaves.
- Add a protein such as grilled chicken or tofu for an even heartier sandwich.

46) LENTIL SOUP

Preparation Time: 10 minutes	**Cooking Time:** 45 minutes	**Servings:** 2

INGREDIENTS:

1 cup dried green or brown lentils, rinsed 1 tablespoon olive oil 1 onion, diced 2 carrots, diced	2 celery stalks, diced 2 garlic cloves, minced 1 teaspoon ground cumin 1/2 teaspoon ground coriander	4 cups vegetable broth 1 can (14 oz) diced tomatoes Salt and pepper to taste

Fresh parsley or cilantro, chopped (for garnish)

INSTRUCTIONS:

1. Heat olive oil in a large pot over medium heat. Add onion, carrots, celery, and garlic. Sauté until the vegetables are softened, about 5 minutes.
2. Stir in the cumin and coriander, cooking for another minute until fragrant.
3. Add the rinsed lentils, vegetable broth, and diced tomatoes (with their juice) to the pot. Bring to a boil.
4. Reduce heat to a simmer, cover, and cook for 35-40 minutes, or until the lentils are tender.
5. Season with salt and pepper to taste. If the soup is too thick, adjust the consistency with additional broth or water.
6. Serve the soup hot, garnished with chopped parsley or cilantro.

NUTRITIONAL VALUES (PER SERVING):

✓ Calories: 380	✓ Fat: 7g	✓ Fiber: 15g
✓ Protein: 22g	✓ Carbohydrates: 60g	

PREPARATION TIPS:

- Soaking lentils beforehand can reduce cooking time and make them easier to digest.
- Use an immersion blender to partially blend the soup for a creamier texture if desired.

SHOPPING TIPS:

- Look for green or brown lentils as they hold their shape well after cooking, providing a pleasing texture to the soup.
- Choose low-sodium vegetable broth to control the salt content of your dish.
- Fresh vegetables should be firm and vibrant in color.

ALTERNATIVE VARIATIONS:

- Add spinach or kale in the last few minutes of cooking for extra greens.
- For a smoky flavor, include a piece of smoked turkey or a sprinkle of smoked paprika.

47) MEDITERRANEAN CHICKPEA SALAD

Preparation Time: 15 minutes	Cooking Time: 0 minutes	Servings: 2

INGREDIENTS:

1 can (15 oz) chickpeas, drained and rinsed	1/4 cup red onion, finely chopped	1 tablespoon lemon juice
1 cucumber, diced	1/4 cup kalamata olives, halved	1 teaspoon dried oregano
1 bell pepper, diced	1/4 cup feta cheese, crumbled	Salt and pepper to taste
	2 tablespoons olive oil	

INSTRUCTIONS:

1. In a large bowl, combine chickpeas, cucumber, bell pepper, red onion, olives, and feta cheese.
2. In a small bowl, whisk together olive oil, lemon juice, oregano, salt, and pepper.
3. Pour the dressing over the salad and toss to combine thoroughly.
4. Adjust seasoning as needed and serve chilled or at room temperature.

NUTRITIONAL VALUES (PER SERVING):

✓ Calories: 350	✓ Fat: 18g	✓ Fiber: 10g
✓ Protein: 12g	✓ Carbohydrates: 38g	

PREPARATION TIPS:

- To enhance the flavors, let the salad marinate in the refrigerator for at least 30 minutes before serving.

SHOPPING TIPS:

- Choose firm cucumbers and bell peppers for the best crunch and freshness.

ALTERNATIVE VARIATIONS:

- For a gluten-free option, ensure all ingredients, especially canned goods, are labeled gluten-free.

48) MEDITERRANEAN CHICKPEA WRAP

Preparation Time: 15 minutes	Cooking Time: 0 minutes	Servings: 2

INGREDIENTS:

1 can (15 oz) chickpeas, rinsed and drained	1/2 cucumber, thinly sliced	1 tablespoon lemon juice
2 large whole wheat tortillas	1/4 red onion, thinly sliced	1 garlic clove, minced
1 cup spinach leaves	1/4 cup feta cheese, crumbled	Salt and pepper to taste
	1/4 cup Greek yogurt	1 teaspoon dried dill (optional)

INSTRUCTIONS:

1. In a small bowl, mix Greek yogurt, lemon juice, minced garlic, salt, pepper, and dill (if using) to make the sauce.
2. Lay out the tortillas and spread each with the yogurt sauce.
3. Down the center of each tortilla, layer spinach leaves, cucumber slices, red onion, chickpeas, and feta cheese.
4. Fold in the sides of the tortilla and roll up tightly to enclose the filling.
5. Cut each wrap in half and serve immediately.

| ✓ Calories: Approximately 400 | ✓ Fat: 10g | ✓ Fiber: 12g |
| ✓ Protein: 20g | ✓ Carbohydrates: 60g | |

PREPARATION TIPS:

- Warm the tortillas slightly to make them more pliable and easier to wrap.
- Adjust the number of garlic and lemon in the yogurt sauce to suit your taste preferences.

SHOPPING TIPS:

- Choose whole wheat tortillas for a healthier option, providing more fiber.
- Look for low-sodium canned chickpeas to reduce your salt intake.

ALTERNATIVE VARIATIONS:

- Add roasted red peppers or olives for extra Mediterranean flavors.
- Substitute chickpeas with grilled chicken or tofu for a different protein choice.

49) PESTO PASTA SALAD

Preparation Time: 15 minutes	**Cooking Time:** 10 minutes	**Servings:** 2

INGREDIENTS:

2 cups cooked pasta (such as fusilli or penne)	1/2 cup pesto sauce (store-bought or homemade) 1 cup cherry tomatoes, halved	1/2 cup mini mozzarella balls Salt and pepper to taste Fresh basil leaves, for garnish

INSTRUCTIONS:

1. Cook the pasta according to package instructions until al dente. Rinse under cold water and drain.
2. In a large bowl, combine the cooled pasta with pesto sauce, cherry tomatoes, and mini mozzarella balls. Toss until everything is evenly coated.
3. Season with salt and pepper to taste.
4. Garnish with fresh basil leaves before serving. Serve chilled or at room temperature.

NUTRITIONAL VALUES (PER SERVING):

| ✓ Calories: 550 | ✓ Fat: 25g | ✓ Fiber: 4g |
| ✓ Protein: 20g | ✓ Carbohydrates: 65g | |

PREPARATION TIPS:

- If the pasta salad seems dry, add a little more pesto or a splash of olive oil to moisten.
- Making your pesto sauce allows you to adjust the flavors to your liking.

SHOPPING TIPS:

- When selecting pasta, opt for whole wheat or legume-based varieties for added fiber and protein.
- For the freshest flavor, look for basil pesto in the refrigerated section of the grocery store, or make your own with fresh basil, pine nuts, Parmesan cheese, garlic, and olive oil.

ALTERNATIVE VARIATIONS:

- Add grilled chicken, shrimp, or white beans for extra protein.
- Incorporate additional vegetables like spinach, arugula, or roasted red peppers for more variety and nutrition.

50) QUINOA & ROASTED VEGETABLE BOWL

Preparation Time: 15 minutes (excluding roasting time)	**Cooking Time:** 30 minutes for roasting vegetables	**Servings:** 2

INGREDIENTS:

1 cup quinoa, cooked according to package instructions 2 cups mixed vegetables (e.g., bell peppers, zucchini, carrots, and red onions), chopped	2 tablespoons olive oil 1 lemon, juiced 1 garlic clove, minced 1/4 teaspoon salt 1/4 teaspoon black pepper	2 tablespoons fresh parsley, chopped

INSTRUCTIONS:

1. Preheat the oven to 400°F (200°C). Toss the chopped vegetables with 1 tablespoon olive oil and spread them out on a baking sheet. Roast for about 30 minutes, or until tender and slightly caramelized.
2. In a small bowl, whisk together the lemon juice, remaining olive oil, minced garlic, salt, and pepper to create the dressing.
3. In a serving bowl, combine the cooked quinoa with the roasted vegetables. Drizzle the lemon vinaigrette over the top and toss to combine.
4. Garnish with fresh parsley before serving.

NUTRITIONAL VALUES (PER SERVING):

| ✓ Calories: 320 | ✓ Fat: 14g | ✓ Fiber: 8g |
| ✓ Protein: 9g | ✓ Carbohydrates: 44g | |

PREPARATION TIPS:

• Roast a large batch of vegetables at the start of the week to save time on meal preparation.

• Select a variety of colorful vegetables for a wide range of nutrients.

ALTERNATIVE VARIATIONS:

• Incorporate roasted chickpeas for added protein and crunch.

51) QUINOA SALAD WITH LEMON VINAIGRETTE

Preparation Time: 20 minutes	**Cooking Time:** 15 minutes	**Servings:** 2

INGREDIENTS:

1 cup quinoa, rinsed	1/4 cup red onion, finely chopped	1 teaspoon honey
2 cups water	1/4 cup fresh parsley, chopped	1 garlic clove, minced
1 cup cherry tomatoes, halved	*For the Lemon Vinaigrette:*	Salt and pepper to taste
1 cucumber, diced	1/4 cup olive oil	
1/2 red bell pepper, diced	2 tablespoons lemon juice	

INSTRUCTIONS:

1. In a medium saucepan, bring 2 cups of water to a boil. Add the quinoa, reduce heat to low, cover, and simmer for 15 minutes or until the quinoa is tender and the water is absorbed. Let cool.
2. In a large bowl, combine the cooled quinoa, cherry tomatoes, cucumber, red bell pepper, red onion, and parsley.
3. In a small bowl, whisk together the olive oil, lemon juice, honey, minced garlic, salt, and pepper to create the vinaigrette.
4. Pour the vinaigrette over the salad and toss until everything is well coated.
5. Adjust seasoning as needed and serve the salad chilled or at room temperature.

NUTRITIONAL VALUES (PER SERVING):

✓ Calories: Approximately 420	✓ Fat: 20g	✓ Fiber: 8g
✓ Protein: 12g	✓ Carbohydrates: 52g	

PREPARATION TIPS:

• To add extra flavor to the quinoa, cook it in vegetable broth instead of water.

• Letting the salad sit for a bit after adding the vinaigrette allows the flavors to meld together.

SHOPPING TIPS:

• Quinoa is available in various colors such as white, red, and black; feel free to use any type or a mix for a colorful presentation.

• Choose fresh, ripe vegetables for the best taste and nutritional content.

ALTERNATIVE VARIATIONS:

• Mix in feta cheese or avocado for creaminess.

• Add grilled chicken or chickpeas for additional protein.

52) QUINOA STUFFED BELL PEPPERS

Preparation Time: 20 minutes	**Cooking Time:** 25 minutes	**Servings:** 2

INGREDIENTS:

2 large bell peppers, halved and seeds removed	1/2 cup corn kernels (fresh, canned, or frozen)	1/4 cup shredded cheese (cheddar, mozzarella, or pepper jack)
1 cup cooked quinoa	1/2 cup tomato sauce	Salt and pepper to taste
1/2 cup canned black beans, drained and rinsed	1 teaspoon ground cumin	Fresh cilantro or parsley for garnish
	1/2 teaspoon chili powder	

INSTRUCTIONS:

1. Preheat your oven to 375°F (190°C). Place the bell pepper halves in a baking dish, cut side up.
2. In a bowl, mix the cooked quinoa, black beans, corn, tomato sauce, cumin, chili powder, salt, and pepper.
3. Spoon the quinoa mixture into each bell pepper half, packing it well.
4. Sprinkle shredded cheese over the top of each stuffed pepper.
5. Cover the baking dish with foil and bake for about 20-25 minutes, or until the peppers are tender and the cheese is bubbly.
6. Garnish with fresh cilantro or parsley before serving.

NUTRITIONAL VALUES (PER SERVING):

✓ Calories: Approximately 350	✓ Fat: 9g	✓ Fiber: 10g
✓ Protein: 15g	✓ Carbohydrates: 55g	

PREPARATION TIPS:

• For a crispier top, remove the foil in the last 5 minutes of baking.

• Adding a splash of lime juice to the quinoa mixture can brighten up the flavors.

SHOPPING TIPS:

• Select bell peppers that are large and have a flat bottom so they can stand up in the baking dish.

• When buying quinoa, look for pre-rinsed varieties to save time on preparation.

ALTERNATIVE VARIATIONS:

- For a non-vegetarian version, add ground turkey or beef to the quinoa mixture.
- Make it vegan by substituting the cheese with a dairy-free cheese alternative or nutritional yeast for a cheesy flavor.

53)   QUINOA TABBOULEH

Preparation Time: 20 minutes	**Cooking Time:** 15 minutes (for quinoa)	**Servings:** 2

INGREDIENTS:

1 cup quinoa, rinsed 2 cups water 1 cup fresh parsley, finely chopped	1/2 cup fresh mint, finely chopped 2 medium tomatoes, diced 1 cucumber, diced	Juice of 2 lemons 2 tablespoons extra-virgin olive oil Salt and pepper to taste

INSTRUCTIONS:

1. In a medium saucepan, combine the quinoa and water. Bring to a boil, then reduce heat to low, cover, and simmer for about 15 minutes, or until the water is absorbed and the quinoa is tender. Allow to cool to room temperature.
2. In a large bowl, combine the cooked quinoa, parsley, mint, tomatoes, and cucumber.
3. In a small bowl, whisk together the lemon juice, olive oil, salt, and pepper to create the dressing.
4. Pour the dressing over the quinoa mixture and toss well to combine.
5. Adjust the seasoning to taste, adding more lemon juice or salt if needed.
6. Serve the tabbouleh chilled or at room temperature.

NUTRITIONAL VALUES (PER SERVING):

✓ Calories: 320 ✓ Protein: 12g	✓ Fat: 10g ✓ Carbohydrates: 49g	✓ Fiber: 8g

PREPARATION TIPS:

- Letting the quinoa cool before mixing it with the herbs and vegetables will prevent the greens from wilting.
- Quinoa tabbouleh can be made in advance and stored in the refrigerator, making it a great option for meal prep.

SHOPPING TIPS:

- Purchase pre-rinsed quinoa to save time or ensure to rinse it well to remove the saponin coating, which can give a bitter taste.
- For the freshest herbs, look for bright, vibrant leaves without any signs of wilting or browning.

ALTERNATIVE VARIATIONS:

- Add chickpeas or feta cheese for extra protein and flavor.
- For a twist, substitute lemon juice with lime juice and olive oil with avocado oil.

54)   ROASTED BUTTERNUT SQUASH SOUP

Preparation Time: 20 minutes	**Cooking Time:** 60 minutes	**Servings:** 2

INGREDIENTS:

1 medium butternut squash, peeled, seeded, and cubed 2 tablespoons olive oil Salt and pepper to taste	1 small onion, diced 2 garlic cloves, minced 4 cups vegetable broth 1/2 teaspoon ground cinnamon	1/4 teaspoon nutmeg 1/2 cup coconut milk (or heavy cream for a richer soup) Pumpkin seeds for garnish (optional)

INSTRUCTIONS:

1. Preheat the oven to 400°F (200°C). Toss the cubed butternut squash with 1 tablespoon olive oil, salt, and pepper. Spread on a baking sheet and roast until tender and caramelized about 25-30 minutes.
2. In a large pot, heat the remaining olive oil over medium heat. Add the diced onion and garlic, sautéing until soft and translucent.
3. Add the roasted butternut squash to the pot along with vegetable broth, cinnamon, and nutmeg. Bring to a boil, then reduce heat and simmer for 20 minutes.
4. Puree the soup using an immersion blender until smooth. Stir in the coconut milk and heat through. Adjust seasoning as needed.
5. Serve the soup hot, garnished with pumpkin seeds if desired.

NUTRITIONAL VALUES (PER SERVING):

✓ Calories: Approximately 300 ✓ Protein: 5g	✓ Fat: 15g ✓ Carbohydrates: 40g	✓ Fiber: 6g

PREPARATION TIPS:

- Roasting the squash before adding it to the soup enhances its sweet, nutty flavor.
- For a smoother texture, pass the pureed soup through a fine sieve.

SHOPPING TIPS:

- Select a firm, heavy butternut squash with a solid beige color and no soft spots.
- Canned coconut milk can be found in the international aisle; shake well before using.

ALTERNATIVE VARIATIONS:

- Incorporate apples or pears for additional sweetness and complexity.
- Garnish with crème fraîche, toasted pecans, or fresh herbs for added flavor and texture.

55) ROASTED VEGETABLE BUDDHA BOWL

Preparation Time: 20 minutes	**Cooking Time:** 30 minutes	**Servings:** 2

INGREDIENTS:

1 sweet potato, peeled and cubed	2 tablespoons olive oil	1 garlic clove, minced
1 cup broccoli florets	Salt and pepper to taste	Water, as needed to thin the dressing
1 red bell pepper, sliced	1 avocado, sliced	Salt to taste
1 cup cooked quinoa	***For the dressing:***	
1 can (15 oz) chickpeas, drained, rinsed, and dried	2 tablespoons tahini	
	1 tablespoon lemon juice	

INSTRUCTIONS:

1. Preheat the oven to 400°F (200°C). Toss the sweet potato, broccoli, and red bell pepper with olive oil, salt, and pepper. Spread on a baking sheet in a single layer.
2. Roast the vegetables in the oven for about 25-30 minutes or until tender and caramelized, turning halfway through.
3. On a separate baking sheet, spread the chickpeas and roast for 20 minutes until crispy.
4. Prepare the dressing by whisking together tahini, lemon juice, minced garlic, and salt. Add water as needed to achieve a pourable consistency.
5. Assemble the Buddha bowls by dividing the quinoa, roasted vegetables, crispy chickpeas, and avocado slices between two bowls.
6. Drizzle with the tahini dressing before serving.

NUTRITIONAL VALUES (PER SERVING):

✓ Calories: 600	✓ Fat: 25g	✓ Fiber: 15g
✓ Protein: 18g	✓ Carbohydrates: 80g	

PREPARATION TIPS:

- Roasting vegetables brings out their natural sweetness and adds depth to their flavor.
- Feel free to swap out any of the vegetables based on seasonal availability or personal preference.

SHOPPING TIPS:

- Choose a variety of colorful vegetables for a visually appealing bowl that's packed with different nutrients.
- Tahini can usually be found in the international aisle or with nut butter in most supermarkets.

ALTERNATIVE VARIATIONS:

- Substitute quinoa with brown rice, farro, or any other grain of your choice.
- For added protein, top the bowl with grilled chicken, tofu, or a boiled egg.

56) SALMON AVOCADO SALAD

Preparation Time: 15 minutes	**Cooking Time:** 10 minutes	**Servings:** 2

INGREDIENTS:

2 salmon fillets (about 6 oz each)	1 avocado, sliced	1 tablespoon lemon juice
Salt and pepper to taste	1/2 cucumber, sliced	1 teaspoon Dijon mustard
1 tablespoon olive oil	1/4 red onion, thinly sliced	1 garlic clove, minced
4 cups mixed greens (such as arugula, spinach, and romaine)	***For the lemon vinaigrette:***	Salt and pepper to taste
	3 tablespoons olive oil	

INSTRUCTIONS:

1. Season the salmon fillets with salt and pepper. Heat olive oil in a skillet over medium-high heat and cook the salmon for about 5 minutes on each side, or until it flakes easily with a fork. Let it cool slightly, then flake into large pieces.
2. In a large bowl, toss the mixed greens, avocado slices, cucumber, and red onion.
3. Prepare the lemon vinaigrette by whisking together olive oil, lemon juice, Dijon mustard, minced garlic, salt, and pepper in a small bowl.
4. Drizzle the vinaigrette over the salad and gently toss to combine.
5. Divide the salad among plates and top with flaked salmon.

NUTRITIONAL VALUES (PER SERVING):

✓ Calories: Approximately 500	✓ Fat: 35g	✓ Fiber: 7g
✓ Protein: 35g	✓ Carbohydrates: 15g	

PREPARATION TIPS:

- Cooking the salmon with its skin on helps keep it moist; you can remove the skin easily after cooking.
- Letting the salad dressing sit for a few minutes before adding it to the salad can enhance its flavors.

SHOPPING TIPS:

- Look for fresh or frozen salmon fillets with vibrant color and firm texture.
- Choose ripe but firm avocados for the best texture in the salad.

ALTERNATIVE VARIATIONS:

- Swap salmon for grilled chicken or tofu for a different protein option.

• Add cherry tomatoes, olives, or capers for extra flavors and textures.

57) SPICY SHRIMP TACOS

Preparation Time: 20 minutes	**Cooking Time:** 10 minutes	**Servings:** 2

INGREDIENTS:

12 large shrimp, peeled and deveined	1/2 teaspoon ground cumin	1/4 cup fresh cilantro, chopped
1 tablespoon olive oil	Salt and pepper to taste	Lime wedges for serving
1 teaspoon chili powder	4 small tortillas (corn or flour)	Optional toppings: avocado slices, sour
1/2 teaspoon garlic powder	1 cup shredded cabbage	cream, salsa

INSTRUCTIONS:

1. In a bowl, toss the shrimp with olive oil, chili powder, garlic powder, cumin, salt, and pepper until well coated.
2. Heat a skillet over medium-high heat. Add the shrimp and cook for 2-3 minutes on each side, or until they are pink and opaque.
3. Warm the tortillas in a dry skillet or directly over a gas flame until soft and pliable.
4. Assemble the tacos by placing a few shrimp on each tortilla, then topping with shredded cabbage and chopped cilantro.
5. Serve with lime wedges and any additional toppings you like.

NUTRITIONAL VALUES (PER SERVING):

✓ Calories: Approximately 400	✓ Fat: 20g	✓ Fiber: 5g
✓ Protein: 25g	✓ Carbohydrates: 35g	

PREPARATION TIPS:

• Marinating the shrimp for 15-30 minutes before cooking can enhance the flavors.

• For extra crispy tortillas, briefly fry them in a bit of oil before assembling the tacos.

SHOPPING TIPS:

• Buy fresh or frozen shrimp; if using frozen, ensure they are thoroughly thawed before cooking.

• Look for high-quality, fresh tortillas – corn tortillas are traditional, but flour tortillas can be used for a softer texture.

ALTERNATIVE VARIATIONS:

• For a vegetarian option, substitute shrimp with grilled vegetables or black beans.

• Add a quick homemade salsa or guacamole for extra freshness and flavor.

58) SWEET POTATO AND BLACK BEAN BURRITOS

Preparation Time: 20 minutes	**Cooking Time:** 25 minutes	**Servings:** 2

INGREDIENTS:

2 medium sweet potatoes, peeled and diced	1/2 teaspoon smoked paprika	1 avocado, sliced
	Salt and pepper to taste	Fresh cilantro, for garnish
1 can (15 oz) black beans, drained and rinsed	4 whole wheat tortillas	Lime wedges, for serving
	1/2 cup grated cheese (cheddar or Monterey Jack)	Optional toppings: sour cream, salsa, diced tomatoes
1 teaspoon ground cumin		

INSTRUCTIONS:

1. Preheat the oven to 400°F (200°C). Toss the sweet potatoes with a bit of olive oil, cumin, smoked paprika, salt, and pepper. Spread on a baking sheet and roast until tender, about 20 minutes.
2. Warm the black beans in a pan and season with a little salt and pepper.
3. Warm the tortillas in the oven or on a skillet to make them pliable.
4. Assemble the burritos: on each tortilla, layer the roasted sweet potatoes, black beans, grated cheese, and avocado slices.
5. Fold in the sides of the tortilla and roll up tightly.
6. Serve the burritos with fresh cilantro, lime wedges, and any additional toppings as desired.

NUTRITIONAL VALUES (PER SERVING):

✓ Calories: Approximately 600	✓ Fat: 25g	✓ Fiber: 15g
✓ Protein: 20g	✓ Carbohydrates: 80g	

PREPARATION TIPS:

• Roasting the sweet potatoes enhances their natural sweetness and complements the savory black beans.

• For a crispy finish, place the assembled burritos back in the oven or on a skillet until the tortillas are golden and the cheese is melted.

SHOPPING TIPS:

• Select firm, orange-fleshed sweet potatoes for the best flavor and texture.

• Whole wheat tortillas are a healthier option, providing additional fiber.

ALTERNATIVE VARIATIONS:

• For a vegan version, omit the cheese or use a dairy-free alternative.

• Add sautéed bell peppers and onions for extra flavor and nutrition.

59) TOMATO BASIL SOUP WITH CHICKPEA CROUTONS

Preparation Time: 10 minutes	**Cooking Time:** 30 minutes	**Servings:** 2

INGREDIENTS:

4 cups ripe tomatoes, chopped	1 tablespoon olive oil	1 tablespoon olive oil
1 onion, finely chopped	Salt and pepper to taste	1/2 teaspoon paprika
2 cloves garlic, minced	***For Chickpea Croutons:***	Salt to taste
2 cups vegetable broth	1 cup canned chickpeas, drained, rinsed,	
1/4 cup fresh basil, chopped	and dried	

INSTRUCTIONS:

1. In a large pot, heat 1 tablespoon olive oil over medium heat. Add the onion and garlic, and sauté until soft.
2. Add the chopped tomatoes and vegetable broth. Bring to a boil, then reduce heat and simmer for 20 minutes.
3. While the soup simmers, preheat the oven to 400°F (200°C). Toss chickpeas with 1 tablespoon olive oil, paprika, and salt. Spread on a baking sheet and bake for 20-25 minutes until crispy.
4. Blend the soup until smooth using an immersion blender. Stir in the chopped basil and season with salt and pepper.
5. Serve the soup hot, topped with crispy chickpea croutons.

NUTRITIONAL VALUES (PER SERVING):

✓ Calories: 250	✓ Fat: 14g	✓ Fiber: 8g
✓ Protein: 7g	✓ Carbohydrates: 28g	

PREPARATION TIPS:

- For a creamier soup, add a splash of coconut milk before blending.

SHOPPING TIPS:

- Choose tomatoes that are deeply colored and firm, with a slightly soft texture for the best flavor.

ALTERNATIVE VARIATIONS:

- Add roasted red peppers to the soup for a smoky flavor or use canned tomatoes for convenience.

60) *TUNA SALAD STUFFED AVOCADOS*

Preparation Time: 10 minutes	**Cooking Time:** 0 minutes	**Servings:** 2

INGREDIENTS:

1 can (5 oz) tuna in water, drained	1 tablespoon Dijon mustard	Salt and pepper to taste
2 ripe avocados, halved and pitted	1/4 cup red onion, finely chopped	Lemon wedges for serving
1/4 cup mayonnaise or Greek yogurt	1/4 cup celery, finely chopped	Fresh dill or parsley for garnish (optional)

INSTRUCTIONS:

1. In a bowl, mix the tuna, mayonnaise (or Greek yogurt), Dijon mustard, red onion, and celery. Season with salt and pepper to taste.
2. Scoop out some of the avocado flesh to create a larger cavity and chop the removed avocado to add to the tuna mixture.
3. Fill the avocado halves with the tuna salad.
4. Serve with lemon wedges on the side and garnish with fresh dill or parsley if desired.

NUTRITIONAL VALUES (PER SERVING):

✓ Calories: Approximately 400	✓ Fat: 30g	✓ Fiber: 13g
✓ Protein: 25g	✓ Carbohydrates: 17g	

PREPARATION TIPS:

- For a lighter version, use Greek yogurt instead of mayonnaise.
- Adding a squeeze of lemon juice to the tuna salad enhances the flavors and adds a fresh zing.

SHOPPING TIPS:

- Select tuna packed in water for a healthier option and to avoid extra oil. Look for brands that are certified sustainable.
- When choosing avocados, go for ones that are just ripe; they should yield slightly to pressure but not be overly soft.

ALTERNATIVE VARIATIONS:

- Substitute tuna with cooked chicken breast or chickpeas for a different protein option.
- Add diced cucumber or chopped tomatoes to the tuna mixture for extra crunch and freshness.

61) *TURKEY AND SPINACH WRAP*

Preparation Time: 10 minutes	**Cooking Time:** 0 minutes	**Servings:** 2

INGREDIENTS:

2 whole grain wraps	1 cup fresh spinach leaves	2 tablespoons hummus
4 slices of turkey breast	1/4 cup shredded carrots	Salt and pepper to taste

INSTRUCTIONS:

1. Lay out the whole-grain wraps on a flat surface.
2. Spread 1 tablespoon of hummus on each wrap.
3. Arrange two slices of turkey breast on each wrap.
4. Top with fresh spinach leaves and shredded carrots.
5. Season with salt and pepper.
6. Roll up the wraps tightly, cut in half, and serve.

✓ Calories: Approximately 300 ✓ Protein: 25g	✓ Fat: 9g ✓ Carbohydrates: 35g	✓ Fiber: 5g

PREPARATION TIPS:

- For added flavor, you can add slices of avocado or a sprinkle of feta cheese.
- Warm the wraps slightly before assembling them to make them more pliable.

SHOPPING TIPS:

- Select whole grain wraps for a healthier option, providing additional fiber and nutrients.
- Look for low-sodium turkey breast slices to keep the wrap healthier.

ALTERNATIVE VARIATIONS:

- Vegetarians can substitute turkey with sliced, grilled tofu or a veggie patty.
- Try different spreads like avocado or tzatziki for a new flavor profile.

62) VEGETABLE STIR-FRY WITH BROWN RICE

Preparation Time: 15 minutes	**Cooking Time:** 20 minutes	**Servings:** 2

INGREDIENTS:

1 cup brown rice 2 cups water 1 tablespoon sesame oil	2 cups mixed vegetables (e.g., bell peppers, broccoli, snap peas, carrots), sliced 2 garlic cloves, minced 1 tablespoon ginger, minced	2 tablespoons soy sauce 1 tablespoon oyster sauce (optional) 1 teaspoon honey (optional) Sesame seeds, for garnish Green onions, sliced, for garnish

INSTRUCTIONS:

1. Rinse the brown rice under cold water until the water runs clear. Combine the rice and water in a pot and bring to a boil. Reduce heat to low, cover, and simmer for about 45 minutes, or until the rice is cooked and water is absorbed.
2. While the rice is cooking, heat sesame oil in a large skillet or wok over medium-high heat. Add the mixed vegetables, garlic, and ginger. Stir-fry for 5-7 minutes, or until the vegetables are tender but still crisp.
3. Stir in the soy sauce, oyster sauce, and honey (if using), coating the vegetables evenly. Cook for an additional 2 minutes.
4. Serve the vegetable stir-fry over the cooked brown rice. Garnish with sesame seeds and green onions.

NUTRITIONAL VALUES (PER SERVING):

✓ Calories: Approximately 350 ✓ Protein: 8g	✓ Fat: 7g ✓ Carbohydrates: 64g	✓ Fiber: 8g

PREPARATION TIPS:

- Cutting vegetables into uniform sizes ensures they cook evenly.
- For added protein, consider tossing in tofu, chicken, or shrimp with the vegetables.

SHOPPING TIPS:

- Opt for fresh, seasonal vegetables for the best flavor and nutritional value.
- Brown rice can be found in the grains section; choose short or long grains depending on your texture preference.

ALTERNATIVE VARIATIONS:

- Swap brown rice for quinoa or cauliflower rice for a different grain base.
- Experiment with different sauces like teriyaki or sweet chili for variety.

Chapter 9.
SNACK RECIPES

---

63)   ALMONDS AND DARK CHOCOLATE

Preparation Time: 5 minutes	**Cooking Time:** 0 minutes	**Servings:** 2

INGREDIENTS:

1/4 cup almonds	1/4 cup dark chocolate pieces

INSTRUCTIONS:

1.Measure out the almonds and dark chocolate pieces.
2.Combine in a small bowl or container for a ready-to-enjoy snack.

NUTRITIONAL VALUES (PER SERVING):

✓ Calories: Approximately 220	✓ Fat: 16g	✓ Fiber: 3g
✓ Protein: 5g	✓ Carbohydrates: 18g	

PREPARATION TIPS:

• For added health benefits, choose dark chocolate with a high cocoa content (70% or higher).
• Roasting the almonds before mixing with chocolate can enhance their flavor.

SHOPPING TIPS:

• Select raw or dry-roasted almonds without added salt for a healthier option.
• Look for dark chocolate that contains minimal added sugar and no artificial ingredients.

ALTERNATIVE VARIATIONS:

• Mix in dried fruit like cherries or cranberries for added sweetness and texture.
• Use a mix of nuts for variety, including walnuts and pecans along with the almonds.

---

64)   APPLE AND PEANUT BUTTER

Preparation Time: 5 minutes	**Cooking Time:** 0 minutes	**Servings:** 2

INGREDIENTS:

1 large apple, cored and sliced	2 tablespoons peanut butter

INSTRUCTIONS:

1.Slice the apple into thin wedges.
2.Serve each portion of apple slices with a tablespoon of peanut butter for dipping.

NUTRITIONAL VALUES (PER SERVING):

✓ Calories: Approximately 280	✓ Fat: 16g	✓ Fiber: 5g
✓ Protein: 8g	✓ Carbohydrates: 30g	

PREPARATION TIPS:

• To prevent the apple slices from browning, you can lightly toss them in a bit of lemon juice.
• Warming the peanut butter slightly can make it easier to dip.

SHOPPING TIPS:

• Choose firm and fresh apples for the best taste and texture. Varieties like Fuji, Gala, or Honeycrisp work well.
• For the healthiest option, select natural peanut butter without added sugars or oils.

ALTERNATIVE VARIATIONS:

• Swap the peanut butter for almond butter or any other nut or seed butter you prefer.
• Sprinkle cinnamon over the apple slices for an added flavor boost.

---

65)   APPLE SLICES WITH ALMOND BUTTER

Preparation Time: 5 minutes	**Cooking Time:** 0 minutes	**Servings:** 2

INGREDIENTS:

2 medium apples, cored and sliced	4 tablespoons almond butter

INSTRUCTIONS:

1.Slice the apples into thin pieces, removing the core.
2.Serve each portion of apple slices with 2 tablespoons of almond butter for dipping.

NUTRITIONAL VALUES (PER SERVING):

✓ Calories: Approximately 280	✓ Fat: 16g	✓ Fiber: 6g
✓ Protein: 6g	✓ Carbohydrates: 34g	

PREPARATION TIPS:

- To prevent the apple slices from browning, you can lightly toss them in lemon juice.
- For a crunchier texture, add a sprinkle of granola or chopped nuts over the almond butter.

SHOPPING TIPS:

- Choose firm apples that have a vibrant color. Varieties like Fuji, Gala, or Honeycrisp are great for snacking.
- Opt for natural almond butter without added sugars or oils for the healthiest option.

ALTERNATIVE VARIATIONS:

- Substitute almond butter with peanut or cashew butter based on your preference.
- Sprinkle cinnamon on the apple slices for an extra flavor boost.

66) APPLE WITH ALMOND BUTTER

Preparation Time: 5 minutes	**Cooking Time:** 0 minutes	**Servings:** 2

INGREDIENTS:

1 large apple, cored and sliced	2 tablespoons almond butter

INSTRUCTIONS:

1. Core and slice the apple into thin pieces.
2. Serve each portion of apple slices with a tablespoon of almond butter for dipping.

NUTRITIONAL VALUES (PER SERVING):

✓ Calories: Approximately 280	✓ Fat: 16g	✓ Fiber: 6g
✓ Protein: 6g	✓ Carbohydrates: 34g	

PREPARATION TIPS:

- To prevent apple slices from browning, you can lightly toss them in lemon juice.
- For a crunchier texture, add a sprinkle of granola or chopped nuts over the almond butter.

SHOPPING TIPS:

- Choose firm apples that have a vibrant color. Varieties like Fuji, Gala, or Honeycrisp are great for snacking.
- Opt for natural almond butter without added sugars or oils for the healthiest option.

ALTERNATIVE VARIATIONS:

- Substitute almond butter with peanut or cashew butter based on your preference.
- Sprinkle cinnamon on the apple slices for an extra flavor boost.

67) CARROT STICKS WITH AVOCADO DIP

Preparation Time: 10 minutes	**Cooking Time:** 0 minutes	**Servings:** 2

INGREDIENTS:

2 large carrots, peeled and cut into sticks	1 lemon, juiced	2 tablespoons cilantro, chopped
1 ripe avocado	1 garlic clove, minced	Salt and pepper to taste

INSTRUCTIONS:

1. In a medium bowl, mash the avocado with a fork until smooth.
2. Stir in lemon juice, minced garlic, cilantro, salt, and pepper until well combined.
3. Serve the avocado dip with carrot sticks on the side for dipping.
4. Enjoy this refreshing and healthy snack immediately.

NUTRITIONAL VALUES (PER SERVING):

✓ Calories: 180	✓ Fat: 14g	✓ Fiber: 7g
✓ Protein: 3g	✓ Carbohydrates: 14g	

PREPARATION TIPS:

- Keep the avocado pit in the dip until serving to help prevent browning.

SHOPPING TIPS:

- Choose carrots that are firm and bright in color. For the avocado, a slightly soft texture indicates ripeness.

ALTERNATIVE VARIATIONS:

- Experiment with adding spices like cumin or paprika to the dip for an extra flavor kick.
- Swap carrots for other vegetables like cucumber or bell pepper sticks for variety.

68) CARROT STICKS WITH HUMMUS

Preparation Time: 5 minutes	**Cooking Time:** 0 minutes	**Servings:** 2

INGREDIENTS:

2 large carrots, peeled and cut into sticks	1/2 cup hummus

INSTRUCTIONS:

1. Peel the carrots and slice them into stick-sized pieces.

2.Serve with hummus for dipping.

NUTRITIONAL VALUES (PER SERVING):

✓ Calories: Approximately 105	✓ Fat: 6g	✓ Fiber: 3g
✓ Protein: 3g	✓ Carbohydrates: 12g	

PREPARATION TIPS:

- Keep the carrots and hummus chilled until ready to serve for a refreshing snack.
- For a variety of flavors and textures, consider adding other vegetables like cucumber or bell pepper sticks.

SHOPPING TIPS:

- Choose firm and bright-colored carrots for the freshest taste and best crunch.
- When selecting hummus, look for options with simple ingredients and without added preservatives.

ALTERNATIVE VARIATIONS:

- Spice up your hummus by adding a sprinkle of paprika or drizzle of olive oil on top.
- Try different hummus flavors like roasted red pepper or garlic for variety.

69) CELERY STICKS WITH ALMOND BUTTER

Preparation Time: 5 minutes	Cooking Time: 0 minutes	Servings: 2

INGREDIENTS:

4 celery stalks, washed and cut into sticks	2 tablespoons almond butter

INSTRUCTIONS:

1.Spread almond butter on each celery stick.
2.Enjoy the crunchy and creamy textures together.

NUTRITIONAL VALUES (PER SERVING):

✓ Calories: Approximately 180	✓ Fat: 15g	✓ Fiber: 3g
✓ Protein: 5g	✓ Carbohydrates: 8g	

PREPARATION TIPS:

- For a variety in texture and flavor, consider adding raisins or dried cranberries on top of the almond butter, creating a "ants on a log" snack.
- If the almond butter is too thick, stir in a teaspoon of coconut oil to make it easier to spread.

SHOPPING TIPS:

- Look for natural almond butter that doesn't contain added sugars or hydrogenated oils.
- Choose celery that is crisp and bright green, with no signs of wilting.

ALTERNATIVE VARIATIONS:

- Swap almond butter for peanut butter, cashew butter, or any nut or seed butter of your preference.
- Sprinkle the almond butter with a dash of cinnamon or cocoa powder for an extra flavor twist.

70) CHEESE AND WHOLE GRAIN CRACKERS

Preparation Time: 5 minutes	Cooking Time: 0 minutes	Servings: 2

INGREDIENTS:

2 ounces cheese (choose your favorite variety)	10 whole grain crackers

INSTRUCTIONS:

1.Cut or slice the cheese into small pieces that fit easily on the crackers.
2.Arrange the cheese and crackers on a plate for easy snacking.

NUTRITIONAL VALUES (PER SERVING):

✓ Calories: Approximately 250	✓ Fat: 15g	✓ Fiber: 3g
✓ Protein: 10g	✓ Carbohydrates: 20g	

PREPARATION TIPS:

- For extra flavor, add a slice of tomato or cucumber on top of the cheese before placing it on the cracker.
- Soft cheeses like brie or goat cheese can be spread directly onto the crackers.

SHOPPING TIPS:

- When selecting cheese, consider varieties that are rich in flavor so you can use less and still be satisfied.
- Look for whole-grain crackers that list whole-grain as the first ingredient for the best nutritional value.

ALTERNATIVE VARIATIONS:

- Vegan or dairy-free? Many plant-based cheeses pair wonderfully with whole-grain crackers.
- Mix up the flavors by choosing different types of cheese and crackers or add a small dollop of jam or honey on top of the cheese for a sweet contrast.

71) COTTAGE CHEESE WITH PINEAPPLE

Preparation Time: 5 minutes	**Cooking Time:** 0 minutes	**Servings:** 2

INGREDIENTS:

1 cup cottage cheese	1/2 cup pineapple chunks

INSTRUCTIONS:

1. Divide the cottage cheese between two bowls.
2. Top each bowl with pineapple chunks.
3. Mix gently and serve for a refreshing and filling snack.

NUTRITIONAL VALUES (PER SERVING):

✓ Calories: Approximately 180	✓ Fat: 5g	✓ Fiber: 1g
✓ Protein: 14g	✓ Carbohydrates: 20g	

PREPARATION TIPS:

- For a smoother texture, blend the cottage cheese before adding the pineapple.
- Chilling both the cottage cheese and pineapple before serving makes this snack even more refreshing.

SHOPPING TIPS:

- Select small-curd, low-fat cottage cheese for a lighter option.
- Fresh pineapple can be substituted with canned pineapple chunks in juice (not syrup) for convenience.

ALTERNATIVE VARIATIONS:

- Sprinkle with toasted coconut flakes or chopped nuts for added texture and flavor.
- Mix in other fruits like mango or berries for a varied fruit profile.

72) COTTAGE CHEESE WITH SLICED PEACHES

Preparation Time: 5 minutes	**Cooking Time:** 0 minutes	**Servings:** 2

INGREDIENTS:

1 cup cottage cheese	1 large peach, sliced

INSTRUCTIONS:

1. Divide the cottage cheese between two bowls.
2. Top with fresh peach slices.
3. Serve immediately, enjoying the blend of creamy texture and sweet, fruity flavors.

NUTRITIONAL VALUES (PER SERVING):

✓ Calories: Approximately 150	✓ Fat: 2g	✓ Fiber: 2g
✓ Protein: 14g	✓ Carbohydrates: 20g	

PREPARATION TIPS:

- If peaches are not in season, canned peaches in juice (not syrup) can be a good alternative. Be sure to drain them well before use.
- For a richer flavor, drizzle a bit of honey or maple syrup over the top.

SHOPPING TIPS:

- Look for ripe peaches that are firm yet slightly soft to the touch for the best flavor.
- Cottage cheese comes in various fat contents. Choose one that fits your dietary preferences, from non-fat to full-fat versions.

ALTERNATIVE VARIATIONS:

- Swap peaches for any other fresh fruit like berries, sliced bananas, or nectarines for variety.
- Add a sprinkle of granola or chopped nuts to add a crunchy texture to the snack.

73) CRUNCHY KALE AND APPLE SALAD

Preparation Time: 15 minutes	**Cooking Time:** 0 minutes	**Servings:** 2

INGREDIENTS:

4 cups of kale, stems removed, and leaves chopped	1/4 cup dried cranberries	1 teaspoon honey
1 large apple, cored and thinly sliced	2 tablespoons goat cheese, crumbled	Salt and pepper to taste
1/4 cup walnuts, roughly chopped	2 tablespoons olive oil	
	1 tablespoon apple cider vinegar	

INSTRUCTIONS:

1. In a large bowl, massage the kale with olive oil and a pinch of salt for about 2 minutes until the leaves start to soften.
2. Add the sliced apple, walnuts, and dried cranberries to the bowl.
3. In a small bowl, whisk together apple cider vinegar, honey, salt, and pepper to make the dressing.
4. Drizzle the dressing over the salad and toss to combine.
5. Top with crumbled goat cheese before serving.

NUTRITIONAL VALUES (PER SERVING):

✓ Calories: 320	✓ Fat: 22g	✓ Fiber: 5g
✓ Protein: 6g	✓ Carbohydrates: 29g	

PREPARATION TIPS:

• Massage kale with a bit of olive oil to soften the leaves and make them easier to digest.

• Look for firm, bright green kale leaves and a crisp apple for the best texture and flavor.

ALTERNATIVE VARIATIONS:

• Swap walnuts with almonds or pecans, and goat cheese with feta or blue cheese for different flavor profiles.

74) CUCUMBER HUMMUS BITES

Preparation Time: 10 minutes	**Cooking Time:** 0 minutes	**Servings:** 2

INGREDIENTS:

1 large cucumber, sliced into rounds 1/2 cup hummus	1/4 cup cherry tomatoes, halved 1 tablespoon fresh parsley, chopped	Pinch of paprika Salt and pepper to taste

INSTRUCTIONS:

1. Arrange cucumber slices on a plate.
2. Spoon a small amount of hummus onto each cucumber round.
3. Top each with a cherry tomato half and sprinkle with chopped parsley.
4. Dust lightly with paprika and season with salt and pepper to taste.
5. Serve immediately or chill for a refreshing snack.

NUTRITIONAL VALUES (PER SERVING):

✓ Calories: 120 ✓ Protein: 6g	✓ Fat: 7g ✓ Carbohydrates: 12g	✓ Fiber: 3g

PREPARATION TIPS:

• For a smoother hummus spread, let the hummus come to room temperature before assembling the bites.

SHOPPING TIPS:

• Choose firm, medium-sized cucumbers for the best bite-sized rounds.

ALTERNATIVE VARIATIONS:

• Experiment with flavored hummus varieties or add a slice of olive for an extra Mediterranean twist.

75) DARK CHOCOLATE AND BERRIES

Preparation Time: 5 minutes	**Cooking Time:** 0 minutes	**Servings:** 2

INGREDIENTS:

2 ounces of dark chocolate (70% cocoa or higher)	1 cup of mixed berries (such as strawberries, blueberries, and raspberries)

INSTRUCTIONS:

1. Break the dark chocolate into small pieces and melt in a microwave-safe bowl in 30-second intervals, stirring until smooth. Alternatively, melt the chocolate in a double boiler over low heat, stirring continuously.
2. Arrange the mixed berries on a plate.
3. Drizzle the melted dark chocolate over the berries or dip the berries into the chocolate and place them on a parchment-lined tray to set.
4. Allow the chocolate to harden slightly before serving or enjoy immediately for a softer chocolate coating.

NUTRITIONAL VALUES (PER SERVING):

✓ Calories: Approximately 200 ✓ Protein: 3g	✓ Fat: 12g ✓ Carbohydrates: 24g	✓ Fiber: 4g

PREPARATION TIPS:

• To enhance the flavor, add a pinch of sea salt or a sprinkle of chili powder to the melted chocolate before drizzling or dipping.
• For a fun variation, freeze the chocolate-covered berries for a refreshing summer treat.

SHOPPING TIPS:

• Look for high-quality dark chocolate with a cocoa content of 70% or higher for the best taste and health benefits.
• Choose fresh, ripe berries for the best flavor and texture. If out of season, frozen berries can be used but thaw and drain them first to avoid excess moisture.

ALTERNATIVE VARIATIONS:

• Substitute dark chocolate with yogurt for a lighter version. Simply mix Greek yogurt with a touch of honey and dip the berries.
• Mix in nuts or seeds with the berries before drizzling with chocolate for added crunch and nutrition.

76) DARK CHOCOLATE SQUARE

Preparation Time: 1 minute	**Cooking Time:** 0 minutes	**Servings:** 2

INGREDIENTS:

2 squares of high-quality dark chocolate (70% cocoa or higher)

INSTRUCTIONS:

1.Break the dark chocolate into individual squares.
2.Serve each square on a small plate or napkin as a rich, decadent snack.

NUTRITIONAL VALUES (PER SERVING):

| ✓ Calories: Approximately 60 | ✓ Fat: 4g | ✓ Fiber: 2g |
| ✓ Protein: 1g | ✓ Carbohydrates: 6g | |

PREPARATION TIPS:

- To fully enjoy the flavor of dark chocolate, let it melt slowly in your mouth rather than chewing it quickly. This allows you to savor the complexity and richness of the chocolate.
- Pairing dark chocolate with a cup of coffee or red wine can enhance its flavors and make for a more sophisticated snack experience.

SHOPPING TIPS:

- When selecting dark chocolate, look for bars with a higher percentage of cocoa (70% or above) as they contain more antioxidants and less sugar.
- Check the ingredients list for minimal additives. High-quality dark chocolate should contain primarily cocoa mass, cocoa butter, and a sweetener.

ALTERNATIVE VARIATIONS:

- For an added crunch, choose dark chocolate with nuts or cacao nibs.
- If you're adventurous, try dark chocolate with unusual flavor pairings like sea salt, chili, or lavender for a unique tasting experience.

77) EDAMAME

| **Preparation Time:** 2 minutes | **Cooking Time:** 5 minutes | **Servings:** 2 |

INGREDIENTS:

| 1 cup edamame, fresh or frozen | Salt to taste |

INSTRUCTIONS:

1.Bring a pot of water to a boil. Add the edamame and cook for about 5 minutes, or just until tender.
2.Drain the edamame and sprinkle with a little salt to taste.
3.Serve warm or at room temperature, enjoying the beans by popping them out of their pods.

NUTRITIONAL VALUES (PER SERVING):

| ✓ Calories: Approximately 100 | ✓ Fat: 4g | ✓ Fiber: 4g |
| ✓ Protein: 8g | ✓ Carbohydrates: 9g | |

PREPARATION TIPS:

- For an added flavor twist, try sprinkling the edamame with chili powder or garlic salt instead of plain salt.
- To eat, simply squeeze the beans out of the pods directly into your mouth. Remember, the pods are not meant to be eaten.

SHOPPING TIPS:

- Edamame can usually be found in the frozen section of most grocery stores. Look for bags that allow you to steam the beans right in the microwave for convenience.
- If using fresh edamame, choose pods that are bright green and feel firm to the touch.

ALTERNATIVE VARIATIONS:

- Drizzle the cooked edamame with a bit of sesame oil and sprinkle with sesame seeds for an Asian-inspired flavor.
- Mix the cooked edamame with a small amount of soy sauce and wasabi for a snack with a kick.

78) FRESH FRUIT SALAD

| **Preparation Time:** 10 minutes | **Cooking Time:** 0 minutes | **Servings:** 2 |

INGREDIENTS:

| 1 cup mixed fresh fruits (berries, melon, kiwi, grapes, etc.) | Optional: A squeeze of fresh lemon or lime juice for added zest |

INSTRUCTIONS:

1.Chop the fruits into bite-sized pieces and mix them in a large bowl.
2.If desired, squeeze a little lemon or lime juice over the fruit salad before serving to enhance the flavors.
3.Serve immediately or chill in the refrigerator for a refreshing snack.

NUTRITIONAL VALUES (PER SERVING):

| ✓ Calories: Varies depending on the fruits used (generally about 100-150 calories) | ✓ Protein: 1-2g
✓ Fat: 0g | ✓ Carbohydrates: 25-35g
✓ Fiber: 3-5g |

PREPARATION TIPS:

- To keep the fruit salad fresh, add a squeeze of citrus juice to prevent browning.
- A sprinkle of chopped fresh mint can add a refreshing twist to the fruit salad.

SHOPPING TIPS:

- Choose a variety of colors and textures of fruit to make the salad more appealing and nutritious.

- Opt for in-season fruits for the best flavor and value.

ALTERNATIVE VARIATIONS:

- For an indulgent twist, drizzle a bit of honey or sprinkle a dash of cinnamon on top of the fruit salad.
- Include a handful of nuts or seeds for a crunchy texture and extra nutrients.

79) FRESH PINEAPPLE CHUNKS

Preparation Time: 10 minutes	**Cooking Time:** 0 minutes	**Servings:** 2

INGREDIENTS:

1/2 fresh pineapple, peeled and cut into chunks

INSTRUCTIONS:

1. Cut the pineapple into bite-sized chunks.
2. Serve the pineapple chunks in small bowls or containers.

NUTRITIONAL VALUES (PER SERVING):

✓ Calories: Approximately 70	✓ Fat: 0g	✓ Fiber: 2g
✓ Protein: 1g	✓ Carbohydrates: 19g	

PREPARATION TIPS:

- To cut the pineapple easily, first slice off the top and bottom. Stand it upright and slice away the skin from top to bottom, then cut it into quarters and remove the core before chopping it into chunks.
- Squeeze a little lime juice over the pineapple chunks to add a zesty flavor.

SHOPPING TIPS:

- A ripe pineapple should have a sweet fragrance at the bottom, bright green leaves, and give slightly to pressure.
- Avoid pineapples with soft spots or bruises, which may indicate over-ripeness or spoilage.

ALTERNATIVE VARIATIONS:

- Combine pineapple chunks with other tropical fruits like mango, kiwi, and papaya for a mixed fruit salad.
- Dip pineapple chunks in melted dark chocolate and refrigerate until the chocolate sets for a decadent treat.

80) GRANOLA BAR

Preparation Time: 15 minutes	**Cooking Time:** 20 minutes	**Servings:** 2

INGREDIENTS:

1 cup rolled oats	1/4 cup dried cranberries or raisins	1 tablespoon melted coconut oil
1/4 cup chopped almonds	2 tablespoons honey or maple syrup	A pinch of salt

INSTRUCTIONS:

1. Preheat the oven to 350°F (175°C). Line a small baking dish with parchment paper.
2. In a bowl, mix the oats, almonds, dried cranberries, honey, coconut oil, and salt.
3. Press the mixture firmly into the prepared baking dish.
4. Bake for 20 minutes or until the edges are golden brown.
5. Let cool completely before cutting into bars.

NUTRITIONAL VALUES (PER SERVING):

✓ Calories: Approximately 300	✓ Fat: 10g	✓ Fiber: 5g
✓ Protein: 6g	✓ Carbohydrates: 50g	

PREPARATION TIPS:

- Press the mixture firmly into the pan to help the bars stick together after baking.
- Allow the bars to cool completely in the pan before slicing to prevent them from falling apart.

SHOPPING TIPS:

- Look for old-fashioned rolled oats for the best texture. Instant oats may become too mushy.
- Choose raw nuts and unsweetened dried fruit to keep added sugars to a minimum.

ALTERNATIVE VARIATIONS:

- Mix in different types of nuts, seeds, or dried fruits to customize the flavor.
- For a chocolatey twist, add dark chocolate chips to the mixture before baking.

81) GREEK YOGURT AND HONEY

Preparation Time: 5 minutes	**Cooking Time:** 0 minutes	**Servings:** 2

INGREDIENTS:

1 cup Greek yogurt	2 tablespoons honey

INSTRUCTIONS:

1. Divide the Greek yogurt into two bowls.
2. Drizzle 1 tablespoon of honey over each serving of yogurt.
3. Stir slightly and enjoy immediately for a creamy, sweet treat.

✓ Calories: Approximately 150	✓ Fat: 0g	✓ Fiber: 0g
✓ Protein: 12g	✓ Carbohydrates: 18g	

PREPARATION TIPS:

- For an added crunch, sprinkle granola or chopped nuts on top of the yogurt before serving.
- If you prefer a bit of tartness, add a squeeze of fresh lemon juice to the yogurt along with the honey.

SHOPPING TIPS:

- Choose plain Greek yogurt to avoid added sugars and flavors, maximizing the health benefits.
- Look for raw, organic honey for its natural flavors and additional health benefits.

ALTERNATIVE VARIATIONS:

- Substitute honey with maple syrup or agave nectar if you're looking for a different type of sweetness.
- Add fresh fruit like berries or sliced bananas for extra vitamins and fiber.

82) GREEK YOGURT WITH CINNAMON

Preparation Time: 5 minutes	**Cooking Time:** 0 minutes	**Servings:** 2

INGREDIENTS:

1 cup Greek yogurt	Optional: honey or maple syrup for
1 teaspoon ground cinnamon	added sweetness

INSTRUCTIONS:

1. Spoon the Greek yogurt into two bowls.
2. Sprinkle the ground cinnamon over the yogurt evenly.
3. Drizzle with honey or maple syrup if desired.
4. Mix lightly and enjoy immediately.

NUTRITIONAL VALUES (PER SERVING):

✓ Calories: Approximately 150	✓ Fat: 0g	✓ Fiber: 0g
✓ Protein: 12g	✓ Carbohydrates: 11g (without honey/maple syrup)	

PREPARATION TIPS:

- For a more decadent snack, add a handful of granolas or chopped nuts for added crunch and flavor.
- To keep your snack interesting, experiment with adding different spices like nutmeg or cardamom alongside cinnamon.

SHOPPING TIPS:

- Opt for plain, unsweetened Greek yogurt to control the amount and type of sweetener used.
- Purchase ground cinnamon or grind your own from cinnamon sticks for the freshest flavor.

ALTERNATIVE VARIATIONS:

- For a vegan alternative, use plant-based yogurt made from coconut, almond, or soy.
- Incorporate fresh fruit such as sliced bananas, apples, or berries for extra sweetness and a boost of vitamins.

83) GREEN ENERGY SMOOTHIE

Preparation Time: 5 minutes	**Cooking Time:** 0 minutes	**Servings:** 2

INGREDIENTS:

1 banana, sliced	1/2 cup unsweetened almond milk	1 teaspoon honey (optional)
1 cup fresh spinach	1 tablespoon chia seeds	

INSTRUCTIONS:

1. Combine all ingredients in a blender.
2. Blend until smooth.
3. Enjoy immediately, topped with a sprinkle of chia seeds.

NUTRITIONAL VALUES (PER SERVING):

✓ Calories: 150	✓ Fat: 4g	✓ Fiber: 5g
✓ Protein: 3g	✓ Carbohydrates: 27g	

PREPARATION TIPS:

- Use frozen banana pieces for an extra-chilled smoothie.

SHOPPING TIPS:

- Opt for dark, richly colored spinach for maximum nutrition.

ALTERNATIVE VARIATIONS:

- Incorporate a scoop of plant-based protein powder for an extra protein kick.

84) HARD-BOILED EGG

Preparation Time: 1 minute	**Cooking Time:** 9-12 minutes	**Servings:** 2

INGREDIENTS:

2 large eggs

INSTRUCTIONS:

1. Place eggs in a saucepan and cover with cold water by an inch.
2. Bring to a boil over medium-high heat, then cover, remove from heat, and let stand for 9-12 minutes.
3. Transfer eggs to a bowl of ice water to cool down quickly.
4. Peel the eggs and serve.

NUTRITIONAL VALUES (PER SERVING):

✓ Calories: Approximately 70 ✓ Protein: 6g	✓ Fat: 5g ✓ Carbohydrates: 1g	✓ Fiber: 0g

PREPARATION TIPS:

• Adding a teaspoon of baking soda to the boiling water can make the eggs easier to peel.
• To ensure even cooking, start with eggs at room temperature.

SHOPPING TIPS:

• Choose eggs that are fresh and free from cracks. Organic or pasture-raised eggs may offer higher nutritional quality.
• Buying eggs in bulk can be more economical, especially if you consume them regularly.

ALTERNATIVE VARIATIONS:

• Sprinkle the eggs with paprika, salt, or your favorite seasoning for added flavor.
• Chop the hard-boiled eggs and mix with a bit of mayonnaise, mustard, and chopped celery for a quick egg salad.

85) HUMMUS AND VEGGIE STICKS

Preparation Time: 10 minutes	**Cooking Time:** 0 minutes	**Servings:** 2

INGREDIENTS:

1/2 cup hummus 1 carrot, peeled and cut into sticks	1 cucumber, cut into sticks 1 bell pepper, cut into sticks	Optional: cherry tomatoes, celery sticks, or any other favorite raw vegetables

INSTRUCTIONS:

1. Clean and prepare the vegetables by cutting them into stick-sized pieces suitable for dipping.
2. Arrange the veggie sticks on a plate or in a serving dish.
3. Place the hummus in a bowl for easy dipping.
4. Enjoy the fresh crunch of vegetables dipped in the rich taste of hummus.

NUTRITIONAL VALUES (PER SERVING):

✓ Calories: Approximately 150 ✓ Protein: 5g	✓ Fat: 9g ✓ Carbohydrates: 13g	✓ Fiber: 4g

PREPARATION TIPS:

• For a homemade touch, consider making your hummus with chickpeas, tahini, lemon juice, and spices blended until smooth.
• To keep the veggies fresh and crisp, store them in water in the refrigerator until ready to serve.

SHOPPING TIPS:

• Select fresh, firm vegetables for the crispiest and most flavorful snack.
• When choosing hummus, look for brands with minimal added oils and preservatives, or opt for making your own for full control over the ingredients.

ALTERNATIVE VARIATIONS:

• Spice up the hummus with additional ingredients such as roasted red peppers, olives, or pine nuts for variety.
• Try different vegetables like radishes, snap peas, or broccoli florets for a diverse nutrient profile.

86) LEMON GARLIC TILAPIA OVER SPINACH

Preparation Time: 5 minutes **Cooking Time:** 12 minutes	**Servings:** 2

INGREDIENTS:

2 tilapia fillets 2 tablespoons olive oil 2 cloves garlic, minced	Juice of 1 lemon 4 cups baby spinach Salt and pepper to taste	Lemon slices and fresh parsley for garnish

INSTRUCTIONS:

1. Preheat the oven to 400°F (200°C).
2. In a small bowl, mix olive oil, garlic, lemon juice, salt, and pepper.
3. Place the tilapia fillets in a baking dish and pour the garlic lemon mixture over them.
4. Bake in the preheated oven for about 12 minutes or until the fish flakes easily with a fork.
5. While the fish is baking, lightly sauté the spinach in a pan with a touch of olive oil until just wilted.
6. Serve the baked tilapia over the wilted spinach, garnished with lemon slices, and chopped parsley.

NUTRITIONAL VALUES (PER SERVING):

<table>
<tr><td>✓ Calories: 280</td><td>✓ Fat: 14g</td><td>✓ Fiber: 1g</td></tr>
<tr><td>✓ Protein: 34g</td><td>✓ Carbohydrates: 3g</td><td></td></tr>
</table>

PREPARATION TIPS:

- For an even more flavorful dish, marinate the tilapia in the garlic-lemon mixture for up to an hour before baking.

SHOPPING TIPS:

- Choose fresh or frozen tilapia fillets based on availability. Look for bright green, fresh spinach leaves for the best taste and nutrition.

ALTERNATIVE VARIATIONS:

- Substitute tilapia with other white fish like cod or haddock. Add cherry tomatoes or capers to the spinach for an extra burst of flavor.

87) MIXED BERRIES

Preparation Time: 5 minutes	**Cooking Time:** 0 minutes	**Servings:** 2

INGREDIENTS:

1/2 cup strawberries, hulled and halved	1/2 cup raspberries
1/2 cup blueberries	1/2 cup blackberries

INSTRUCTIONS:

1. Combine all the berries in a large bowl. Gently toss to mix.
2. Serve the mixed berries in individual bowls or cups for a refreshing snack.

NUTRITIONAL VALUES (PER SERVING):

<table>
<tr><td>✓ Calories: Approximately 70</td><td>✓ Fat: 0.5g</td><td>✓ Fiber: 5g</td></tr>
<tr><td>✓ Protein: 1g</td><td>✓ Carbohydrates: 17g</td><td></td></tr>
</table>

PREPARATION TIPS:

- To enhance the natural sweetness of the berries, let them sit at room temperature for about 10 minutes before serving.
- A drizzle of honey or a sprinkle of chopped fresh mint can add an extra layer of flavor.

SHOPPING TIPS:

- Choose berries that are firm, plump, and deeply colored, avoiding any that are mushy or bruised.
- When berries are out of season, frozen mixed berries can be a convenient and equally nutritious alternative.

ALTERNATIVE VARIATIONS:

- For a creamier snack, serve the mixed berries over Greek yogurt or cottage cheese.
- To add a crunchy texture, sprinkle granola or chopped nuts on top of the berries.

88) MIXED NUTS

Preparation Time: 5 minutes	**Cooking Time:** 0 minutes	**Servings:** 2

INGREDIENTS:

1/2 cup mixed nuts (almonds, walnuts, pecans, cashews)

INSTRUCTIONS:

1. Measure out the mixed nuts into a small bowl or container.
2. Enjoy as is, or lightly toast for enhanced flavor.

NUTRITIONAL VALUES (PER SERVING):

<table>
<tr><td>✓ Calories: Approximately 300</td><td>✓ Fat: 27g</td><td>✓ Fiber: 3g</td></tr>
<tr><td>✓ Protein: 7g</td><td>✓ Carbohydrates: 9g</td><td></td></tr>
</table>

PREPARATION TIPS:

- Toasting nuts in a dry skillet over medium heat until fragrant can deepen their flavor.
- For added spice, toss the nuts with a little cayenne pepper or cinnamon before toasting.

SHOPPING TIPS:

- Look for unsalted, raw, or dry-roasted nuts to keep sodium intake in check.
- Buying nuts in bulk can be more economical and allows for customizing your mix.

ALTERNATIVE VARIATIONS:

- Include seeds like pumpkin or sunflower seeds in your mix for variety.
- For a sweet and salty mix, add a few dried cranberries or dark chocolate chips to the nuts.

89) NUTS AND SEEDS MIX

Preparation Time: 5 minutes	**Cooking Time:** 0 minutes	**Servings:** 2

INGREDIENTS:

1/4 cup almonds	2 tablespoons pumpkin seeds	Optional: a pinch of salt or spice blend
1/4 cup walnuts	2 tablespoons sunflower seeds	for flavoring

INSTRUCTIONS:

1. Combine almonds, walnuts, pumpkin seeds, and sunflower seeds in a bowl.
2. If desired, lightly toast the mixture in a dry pan over medium heat for 3-5 minutes, stirring frequently to prevent burning.

3.Season with a pinch of salt or your favorite spice blend for an extra flavor kick.

4.Let cool and serve as a crunchy, energizing snack.

NUTRITIONAL VALUES (PER SERVING):

✓ Calories: Approximately 300	✓ Fat: 26g	✓ Fiber: 6g
✓ Protein: 10g	✓ Carbohydrates: 12g	

PREPARATION TIPS:

- Roasting the nuts and seeds can enhance their flavor. Spread them on a baking sheet and roast at 350°F (175°C) for 10-15 minutes, stirring occasionally, until they're golden and fragrant.
- Experiment with different combinations of nuts and seeds based on your preferences. Each type brings its own set of nutrients and flavors.

SHOPPING TIPS:

- Bulk bins at grocery stores are a great place to find a variety of nuts and seeds at a lower cost. You can buy exactly the amount you need and try new types without committing to a large package.
- Look for unsalted and unroasted nuts and seeds to control the amount of sodium and ensure they're as natural as possible.

ALTERNATIVE VARIATIONS:

- Spice up your mix with a sprinkle of cayenne pepper, cinnamon, or a dash of soy sauce before roasting for added flavor.
- Add dried fruit like cranberries or chopped apricots to the mix for a touch of sweetness and a chewy texture.

90)   PEACH SLICES WITH COTTAGE CHEESE

Preparation Time: 5 minutes	**Cooking Time:** 0 minutes	**Servings:** 2

INGREDIENTS:

1 large peach, sliced	1 cup cottage cheese

INSTRUCTIONS:

1.Arrange the peach slices on top of the cottage cheese and divide between two bowls.

2.Serve immediately, enjoying the blend of flavors and textures.

NUTRITIONAL VALUES (PER SERVING):

✓ Calories: Approximately 150	✓ Fat: 2g	✓ Fiber: 2g
✓ Protein: 14g	✓ Carbohydrates: 20g	

PREPARATION TIPS:

- For an added flavor boost, drizzle a little honey or sprinkle some cinnamon over the top before serving.
- To keep it chilled and refreshing, ensure both the peach and cottage cheese are served cold.

SHOPPING TIPS:

- Choose ripe peaches for the best sweetness and texture; they should be firm but yield slightly to pressure.
- Opt for low-fat or full-fat cottage cheese based on your dietary preferences; full-fat versions tend to be creamier.

ALTERNATIVE VARIATIONS:

- Substitute peaches with nectarines, apricots, or any seasonal fruit of your choice for different flavors.
- Mix in a handful of nuts or granola for added crunch and nutrition.

91)   PROTEIN SHAKE

Preparation Time: 5 minutes	**Cooking Time:** 0 minutes	**Servings:** 2

INGREDIENTS:

2 scoops protein powder (your choice of flavor) 1 cup almond milk (or any milk of choice)	1/2 banana 1/4 cup mixed berries (fresh or frozen)	Optional: a handful of spinach or a tablespoon of nut butter for added nutrition and flavor

INSTRUCTIONS:

1.Place all ingredients in a blender.

2.Blend on high until smooth and creamy.

3.Adjust the consistency by adding more milk if needed.

4.Pour into glasses and serve immediately for a refreshing and protein-packed snack.

NUTRITIONAL VALUES (PER SERVING):

✓ Calories: Varies depending on protein powder and additional ingredients	✓ Protein: Approximately 20g (varies with protein powder) ✓ Fat: Varies with choice of milk and optional ingredients	✓ Carbohydrates: Varies with fruit and optional ingredients ✓ Fiber: Varies with fruit and optional ingredients

PREPARATION TIPS:

- If using frozen fruit, there's no need to add ice, which makes your shake cold and thick.
- For an extra nutritional boost, consider adding chia seeds or flaxseeds to your shake.

SHOPPING TIPS:

- Choose a high-quality protein powder that meets your dietary preferences and nutritional needs.
- When selecting almond milk or any alternative, opt for unsweetened versions to minimize added sugar.

ALTERNATIVE VARIATIONS:

- Mix up the fruits according to season and preference for different flavors.
- For added texture, top your shake with a sprinkle of granola or coconut flakes.

92) RICE CAKES WITH AVOCADO

Preparation Time: 5 minutes	Cooking Time: 0 minutes	Servings: 2

INGREDIENTS:

2 rice cakes 1 ripe avocado	Salt and pepper to taste	Optional toppings: chili flakes, lemon juice, or sliced tomatoes

INSTRUCTIONS:

1. Mash the ripe avocado in a bowl and season with salt and pepper.
2. Spread the mashed avocado evenly onto the rice cakes.
3. Add any optional toppings as desired for extra flavor.
4. Serve immediately to enjoy the mix of creamy and crunchy textures.

NUTRITIONAL VALUES (PER SERVING):

✓ Calories: Approximately 200 ✓ Protein: 3g	✓ Fat: 15g ✓ Carbohydrates: 15g	✓ Fiber: 7g

PREPARATION TIPS:

- For an extra kick, sprinkle some chili flakes on top of the avocado.
- Adding a squeeze of lemon juice not only enhances the flavor but also helps prevent the avocado from browning.

SHOPPING TIPS:

- Choose firm but ripe avocados; they should give slightly when gently pressed without being too soft.
- Look for whole-grain rice cakes for an added nutritional benefit.

ALTERNATIVE VARIATIONS:

- For a protein boost, consider adding a layer of cottage cheese under the avocado.
- Swap rice cakes for thin slices of whole-grain bread if preferred.

93) SLICED CUCUMBER WITH LIME AND SALT

Preparation Time: 5 minutes	Cooking Time: 0 minutes	Servings: 2

INGREDIENTS:

1 large cucumber, sliced	1 lime, cut into wedges	Salt to taste

INSTRUCTIONS:

1. Arrange the cucumber slices on a plate.
2. Squeeze lime wedges over the cucumber slices to your liking.
3. Season with salt to taste.

NUTRITIONAL VALUES (PER SERVING):

✓ Calories: Approximately 25 ✓ Protein: 1g	✓ Fat: 0g ✓ Carbohydrates: 6g	✓ Fiber: 2g

PREPARATION TIPS:

- For added flavor, sprinkle chili powder or smoked paprika over the cucumbers along with the lime and salt.
- Chill the cucumber in the refrigerator before slicing it for an extra refreshing snack.

SHOPPING TIPS:

- Select cucumbers that are firm and bright green without any yellow spots or blemishes.
- For juicier limes, choose ones that are slightly soft when gently squeezed.

ALTERNATIVE VARIATIONS:

- Swap cucumber for slices of jicama or zucchini for a different but equally refreshing snack.
- Add a drizzle of olive oil or a sprinkle of feta cheese for a Mediterranean twist.

94) TRAIL MIX

Preparation Time: 5 minutes	Cooking Time: 0 minutes	Servings: 2

INGREDIENTS:

1/4 cup almonds 1/4 cup walnuts	2 tablespoons dried cranberries 2 tablespoons pumpkin seeds	1/4 cup dark chocolate chips

INSTRUCTIONS:

1. In a bowl, combine the almonds, walnuts, dried cranberries, pumpkin seeds, and dark chocolate chips.

2.Mix well to evenly distribute the ingredients.

3.Divide the trail mix into two portions for a ready-to-go snack.

NUTRITIONAL VALUES (PER SERVING):

✓ Calories: Approximately 300	✓ Fat: 20g	✓ Fiber: 4g
✓ Protein: 8g	✓ Carbohydrates: 24g	

PREPARATION TIPS:

- Toasting the nuts and seeds in a dry pan over medium heat can enhance their flavor and crunch.
- For a lower sugar option, opt for unsweetened dried fruits and dark chocolate with a high cocoa content.

SHOPPING TIPS:

- Bulk bins are a great resource for purchasing nuts, seeds, and dried fruits as you can buy exactly the amount you need often at a better price than pre-packaged.
- Look for raw or dry-roasted nuts to avoid added oils and salt.

ALTERNATIVE VARIATIONS:

- Customize your trail mix based on your taste preferences and dietary needs. Try adding coconut flakes, and dried apricots, or swap in cashews for almonds.
- For a spicy twist, add a pinch of cayenne pepper or cinnamon to the mix before serving.

95) YOGURT WITH PUMPKIN SEEDS

Preparation Time: 5 minutes	Cooking Time: 0 minutes	Servings: 2

INGREDIENTS:

1 cup plain Greek yogurt	2 tablespoons pumpkin seeds

INSTRUCTIONS:

1.Divide the Greek yogurt between two bowls.

2.Sprinkle pumpkin seeds over the yogurt.

3.Serve immediately, enjoying the creamy and crunchy textures.

NUTRITIONAL VALUES (PER SERVING):

✓ Calories: Approximately 180	✓ Fat: 9g	✓ Fiber: 1g
✓ Protein: 18g	✓ Carbohydrates: 8g	

PREPARATION TIPS:

- To enhance the flavor, lightly toast the pumpkin seeds in a dry skillet over medium heat until they begin to pop.
- Mixing a teaspoon of honey or maple syrup into the yogurt can add a natural sweetness.

SHOPPING TIPS:

- Choose plain Greek yogurt for its higher protein content and lower sugar compared to flavored yogurts.
- Pumpkin seeds are also labeled as pepitas in stores; they can be found in the nuts and seeds section.

ALTERNATIVE VARIATIONS:

- Swap pumpkin seeds for another type of seed or nut, such as sunflower seeds or slivered almonds, to vary the texture and nutrients.
- Add fresh fruits like berries or diced apples for extra sweetness and fiber.

96) GREEK YOGURT AND HONEY WITH WALNUTS

Preparation Time: 5 minutes	Cooking Time: 0 minutes	Servings: 2

INGREDIENTS:

1 cup Greek yogurt (full fat recommended for added creaminess)	2 tablespoons honey 1/4 cup walnuts, roughly chopped	A pinch of cinnamon (optional)

INSTRUCTIONS:

1.Divide the Greek yogurt between two bowls.

2.Drizzle each bowl of yogurt with honey.

3.Sprinkle chopped walnuts over the top of each serving.

4.For a touch of spice, add a pinch of cinnamon to each bowl.

5.Serve immediately and enjoy this wholesome, delicious snack.

NUTRITIONAL INFORMATION (PER SERVING):

✓ Calories: 230	✓ Fat: 12g	✓ Fiber: 1g
✓ Protein: 12g	✓ Carbohydrates: 20g	

PREPARATION TIPS:

- For added texture and flavor, toast the walnuts lightly in a dry pan before adding them to the yogurt.

SHOPPING TIPS:

- Opt for high-quality, full-fat Greek yogurt to maximize the nutritional benefits and ensure a rich, satisfying taste.

ALTERNATIVE VARIATIONS:

- Swap out walnuts for almonds or pecans or add fresh berries or sliced fruit for extra sweetness and a vitamin boost.

Chapter 10.
DINNER RECIPES

97) BAKED COD WITH HERB CRUST

Preparation Time: 10 minutes	Cooking Time: 15 minutes	Servings: 2

INGREDIENTS:

2 cod fillets (about 6 ounces each) 2 tablespoons olive oil 1/2 cup breadcrumbs	2 tablespoons fresh parsley, finely chopped 1 tablespoon fresh thyme leaves 1 garlic clove, minced	Zest of 1 lemon Salt and pepper to taste Lemon wedges for serving

INSTRUCTIONS:

1. Preheat your oven to 400°F (200°C). Line a baking sheet with parchment paper.
2. In a small bowl, mix the breadcrumbs, parsley, thyme, garlic, lemon zest, salt, and pepper.
3. Brush each cod fillet with olive oil, then press the breadcrumb mixture onto the top of each fillet to form a crust.
4. Place the crusted cod fillets on the prepared baking sheet. Bake for about 15 minutes, or until the fish is cooked through and the crust is golden.
5. Serve immediately with lemon wedges on the side.

NUTRITIONAL VALUES (PER SERVING):

✓ Calories: Approximately 320 ✓ Protein: 28g	✓ Fat: 14g ✓ Carbohydrates: 18g	✓ Fiber: 1g

PREPARATION TIPS:

- Ensure the cod fillets are dry by patting them with paper towels before applying the olive oil and breadcrumb mixture. This helps the crust adhere better and become crisper.
- For an even crunchier crust, lightly toast the breadcrumbs in a skillet with a bit of olive oil before mixing them with the herbs and lemon zest.

SHOPPING TIPS:

- Look for fresh or frozen cod fillets with a firm texture and a clean, not fishy, smell.
- Fresh herbs will provide the best flavor for the crust, but dried herbs can be used in a pinch. If using dried, reduce the quantity by half.

ALTERNATIVE VARIATIONS:

- Substitute cod with another white fish like haddock or tilapia, adjusting the cooking time if necessary.
- For a gluten-free version, use gluten-free breadcrumbs or almond flour as a substitute for regular breadcrumbs.

98) BAKED COD WITH ROASTED SWEET POTATOES

Preparation Time: 10 minutes	Cooking Time: 25 minutes	Servings: 2

INGREDIENTS:

2 cod fillets (6 ounces each) 2 sweet potatoes, peeled and diced	2 tablespoons olive oil Salt and pepper to taste	Fresh herbs for garnish (such as parsley or thyme)

INSTRUCTIONS:

1. Preheat your oven to 400°F (200°C). Toss the diced sweet potatoes with 1 tablespoon of olive oil, salt, and pepper. Spread them on a baking sheet and roast for 20-25 minutes, until tender and caramelized.
2. Meanwhile, brush the cod fillets with the remaining olive oil and season with salt and pepper. Place the cod on a lined baking sheet.
3. Bake the cod in the preheated oven for 12-15 minutes or until the fish flakes easily with a fork.
4. Serve the baked cod alongside the roasted sweet potatoes, garnished with fresh herbs.

NUTRITIONAL VALUES (PER SERVING):

✓ Calories: Approximately 350 ✓ Protein: 28g	✓ Fat: 14g ✓ Carbohydrates: 34g	✓ Fiber: 5g

PREPARATION TIPS:

- Ensure the sweet potatoes are cut into even-sized pieces for uniform roasting.
- Pat the cod fillets dry with paper towels before seasoning to help the skin crisp up in the oven.

SHOPPING TIPS:

- Select cod fillets that are moist and have a fresh sea aroma. Avoid fillets that look dry or have a strong fishy smell.
- Choose sweet potatoes that are firm, free of soft spots, and even in color.

ALTERNATIVE VARIATIONS:

- Swap cod for another white fish like haddock or tilapia based on availability and preference.
- Experiment with different seasonings for the sweet potatoes, such as paprika, garlic powder, or cinnamon for a twist.

99) BEEF AND VEGETABLE SKEWERS

Preparation Time: 20 minutes	Cooking Time: 10 minutes	Servings: 2

INGREDIENTS:

1/2 lb. beef (sirloin or tenderloin), cut into 1-inch cubes 1 bell pepper, cut into 1-inch pieces 1 zucchini, sliced into 1/2-inch rounds	1 red onion, cut into 1-inch pieces 2 tablespoons olive oil 2 tablespoons soy sauce 1 garlic clove, minced	1 teaspoon dried oregano Salt and pepper to taste Wooden or metal skewers

INSTRUCTIONS:

1. In a bowl, whisk together olive oil, soy sauce, garlic, oregano, salt, and pepper. Add beef cubes, tossing to coat. Marinate for at least 30 minutes, or up to 2 hours in the refrigerator.
2. Preheat the grill to medium-high heat.
3. Thread the marinated beef, bell pepper, zucchini, and red onion onto skewers.
4. Grill skewers, turning occasionally, until the beef is cooked to your desired level of doneness and the vegetables are tender, about 8-10 minutes.

NUTRITIONAL VALUES (PER SERVING):

✓ Calories: Approximately 400 ✓ Protein: 25g	✓ Fat: 28g ✓ Carbohydrates: 10g	✓ Fiber: 2g

PREPARATION TIPS:

- Soak wooden skewers in water for at least 30 minutes before grilling to prevent them from burning.
- For even cooking, cut the beef and vegetables into similar-sized pieces.

SHOPPING TIPS:

- Choose beef that is well-marbled for the most flavor and tenderness.
- When selecting vegetables, look for bright colors and firm textures, indicating freshness.

ALTERNATIVE VARIATIONS:

- For a vegetarian option, substitute beef with tofu or halloumi cheese.
- Mix and match vegetables based on seasonality and preference. Mushrooms, cherry tomatoes, and eggplant make great additions.

100) BLACK BEAN AND SWEET POTATO TACOS

Preparation Time: 15 minutes	Cooking Time: 25 minutes	Servings: 2

INGREDIENTS:

1 large, sweet potato, peeled and diced 1 tablespoon olive oil 1 teaspoon ground cumin Salt and pepper to taste	1 can (15 oz) black beans, drained and rinsed 4 small corn tortillas	Toppings: avocado slices, diced tomatoes, shredded lettuce, cilantro, lime wedges, and sour cream

INSTRUCTIONS:

1. Preheat your oven to 425°F (220°C). Toss diced sweet potatoes with olive oil, cumin, salt, and pepper. Spread on a baking sheet and roast until tender and slightly caramelized, about 20-25 minutes.
2. Warm the black beans in a saucepan over medium heat, seasoning with additional cumin, salt, and pepper if desired.
3. Warm tortillas according to package instructions.
4. Assemble the tacos by layering roasted sweet potato and black beans onto each tortilla. Add your choice of toppings.
5. Serve immediately with lime wedges on the side for squeezing.

NUTRITIONAL VALUES (PER SERVING):

✓ Calories: Approximately 400 ✓ Protein: 14g	✓ Fat: 12g ✓ Carbohydrates: 64g	✓ Fiber: 17g

PREPARATION TIPS:

- Cutting the sweet potatoes into small, even-sized pieces ensures they roast quickly and evenly.
- For extra crispy sweet potatoes, avoid overcrowding them on the baking sheet.

SHOPPING TIPS:

- Select firm, medium-sized sweet potatoes for the best texture and sweetness.
- Corn tortillas can be found in the international aisle of most supermarkets; look for ones with minimal ingredients for the best flavor.

ALTERNATIVE VARIATIONS:

- For a gluten-free meal, ensure the corn tortillas are certified gluten-free.
- Mix in spices like chili powder or smoked paprika with the sweet potatoes before roasting for additional flavor.

101) CAULIFLOWER STEAK WITH CHIMICHURRI SAUCE

Preparation Time: 15 minutes	Cooking Time: 25 minutes	Servings: 2

INGREDIENTS:

1 large head of cauliflower	*For the Chimichurri Sauce:*	2 tablespoons red wine vinegar
2 tablespoons olive oil	1/2 cup fresh parsley, finely chopped	2 garlic cloves, minced
Salt and pepper to taste	1/4 cup fresh cilantro, finely chopped	1/2 teaspoon red pepper flakes
	1/4 cup olive oil	Salt to taste

INSTRUCTIONS:

1. Preheat the oven to 425°F (220°C).
2. Slice the cauliflower into 1-inch-thick steaks, keeping the stem intact to hold the steaks together.
3. Brush both sides of each cauliflower steak with olive oil and season with salt and pepper. Place on a baking sheet.
4. Roast in the preheated oven for about 25 minutes, flipping halfway through, until tender and golden brown.
5. While the cauliflower roasts, mix all the ingredients for the chimichurri sauce in a bowl. Adjust seasoning as needed.
6. Serve the roasted cauliflower steaks drizzled with chimichurri sauce.

NUTRITIONAL VALUES (PER SERVING):

✓ Calories: Approximately 350	✓ Fat: 31g	✓ Fiber: 5g
✓ Protein: 5g	✓ Carbohydrates: 15g	

PREPARATION TIPS:

- For additional flavor, you can add a sprinkle of smoked paprika or cumin to the cauliflower before roasting.
- Letting the chimichurri sauce sit for a few hours before serving can help meld the flavors together more cohesively.

SHOPPING TIPS:

- Choose a cauliflower head that feels heavy for its size with tightly packed florets and no brown spots.
- Fresh herbs are key for a vibrant and flavorful chimichurri. Ensure they're fresh and not wilted.

ALTERNATIVE VARIATIONS:

- Swap out cauliflower for thick slices of portobello mushrooms or eggplant for a different take on "steak."
- For a spicier chimichurri, increase the amount of red pepper flakes or add a diced jalapeño to the sauce.

102)   CHICKEN AND VEGETABLE SOUP

Preparation Time: 15 minutes	**Cooking Time:** 30 minutes	**Servings:** 2

INGREDIENTS:

2 chicken breasts, diced	2 celery stalks, sliced	1/2 cup frozen peas
1 tablespoon olive oil	4 cups chicken broth	Fresh parsley, chopped, for garnish
1 onion, chopped	1 teaspoon dried thyme	
2 carrots, peeled and sliced	Salt and pepper to taste	

INSTRUCTIONS:

1. In a large pot, heat olive oil over medium heat. Add the diced chicken and cook until no longer pink. Remove chicken and set aside.
2. In the same pot, add onion, carrots, and celery. Cook until the vegetables are softened, about 5 minutes.
3. Return the chicken to the pot and add chicken broth, thyme, salt, and pepper. Bring to a simmer and cook for 20 minutes.
4. Stir in frozen peas and cook for an additional 5 minutes.
5. Adjust seasoning if necessary. Serve hot, garnished with fresh parsley.

NUTRITIONAL VALUES (PER SERVING):

✓ Calories: Approximately 300	✓ Fat: 10g	✓ Fiber: 4g
✓ Protein: 35g	✓ Carbohydrates: 20g	

PREPARATION TIPS:

- For a richer flavor, you can sauté the chicken with a bit of garlic before adding the vegetables.
- Adding the peas towards the end of cooking preserves their bright color and slight crunch.

SHOPPING TIPS:

- Choose fresh, organic vegetables, if possible, for the best flavor and nutrient content.
- If using store-bought chicken broth, look for low-sodium options to control the salt level of the soup.

ALTERNATIVE VARIATIONS:

- Swap out the chicken for turkey or keep it vegetarian by using vegetable broth and adding more legumes like lentils or chickpeas.
- Include other vegetables like potatoes, zucchini, or kale for added nutrition and variety.

103)   CHICKEN STIR-FRY WITH VEGETABLES

Preparation Time: 15 minutes	**Cooking Time:** 10 minutes	**Servings:** 2

INGREDIENTS:

2 boneless, skinless chicken breasts, thinly sliced	1 cup broccoli florets	1 teaspoon ginger, grated
1 bell pepper, julienned	2 tablespoons soy sauce	Salt and pepper to taste
1 carrot, julienned	1 tablespoon sesame oil	Cooked rice, for serving
	1 garlic clove, minced	

INSTRUCTIONS:

1. Heat the sesame oil in a large skillet or wok over medium-high heat. Add the chicken and stir-fry until cooked through, about 5-6 minutes. Remove from the pan and set aside.
2. In the same pan, add the bell pepper, carrot, and broccoli. Stir-fry for 3-4 minutes, or until just tender.
3. Add the garlic and ginger, cooking for an additional minute until fragrant.
4. Return the chicken to the pan. Add the soy sauce and toss everything together until well coated and heated through.
5. Season with salt and pepper to taste. Serve over cooked rice.

NUTRITIONAL VALUES (PER SERVING):

✓ Calories: Approximately 350	✓ Protein: 26g; Fat: 10g ✓ Carbohydrates: 40g	✓ Fiber: 5g

PREPARATION TIPS:

- Cutting the chicken and vegetables into similar-sized pieces ensures they cook evenly.
- For the best flavor, use fresh garlic and ginger rather than powdered.

SHOPPING TIPS:

- Fresh vegetables are ideal, but frozen stir-fry mixes can be a convenient and time-saving option.
- When purchasing chicken, look for cuts that are pinkish and have little to no odor.

ALTERNATIVE VARIATIONS:

- Easily make this dish vegetarian by substituting tofu or tempeh for the chicken.
- Mix in other vegetables like snap peas, mushrooms, or baby corn for more variety and color.

104)   DINNER: ROASTED BUTTERNUT SQUASH AND CHICKPEA CURRY

Preparation Time: 15 minutes	**Cooking Time:** 30 minutes	**Servings:** 2

INGREDIENTS:

2 cups butternut squash, cubed 1 can (15 oz) chickpeas, drained and rinsed 1 tablespoon olive oil	1 onion, diced 2 cloves garlic, minced 1 tablespoon curry powder 1 can (14 oz) coconut milk	2 cups spinach Salt and pepper to taste Fresh cilantro for garnish Cooked brown rice, for serving

INSTRUCTIONS:

1. Preheat the oven to 425°F (220°C). Toss the butternut squash cubes with olive oil, salt, and pepper, and spread them on a baking sheet. Roast for 25 minutes, or until tender and lightly caramelized.
2. In a large skillet, heat a bit more olive oil over medium heat. Sauté the onion and garlic until soft and fragrant.
3. Stir in the curry powder, cooking for another minute until it's well combined with the onions and garlic.
4. Add the roasted butternut squash, chickpeas, and coconut milk to the skillet. Let the curry simmer for 10 minutes, allowing the flavors to meld.
5. Stir in the spinach until it wilts.
6. Serve the curry over cooked brown rice, garnished with fresh cilantro.

NUTRITIONAL VALUES (PER SERVING):

✓ Calories: 495 ✓ Protein: 12g	✓ Fat: 28g ✓ Carbohydrates: 58g	✓ Fiber: 13g

PREPARATION TIPS:

- Roasting the butternut squash before adding it to the curry enhances its sweetness and texture.

SHOPPING TIPS:

- For convenience, opt for pre-cut butternut squash if available.
- Choose a good quality, full-fat coconut milk for the creamiest texture.

ALTERNATIVE VARIATIONS:

- Incorporate additional vegetables like bell peppers or peas for more color and nutrition.
- Swap chickpeas for lentils or tofu for a different protein source.

105)   DINNER: VEGGIE STIR-FRY WITH TOFU

Preparation Time: 15 minutes	**Cooking Time:** 10 minutes	**Servings:** 2

INGREDIENTS:

1 block (14 oz) firm tofu, pressed and cubed 2 cups broccoli florets 1 red bell pepper, sliced	1 carrot, julienned 2 tablespoons soy sauce 1 tablespoon sesame oil 2 garlic cloves, minced	1 tablespoon fresh ginger, grated 1 teaspoon honey (optional) 2 teaspoons sesame seeds 1 tablespoon vegetable oil

INSTRUCTIONS:

1. Heat vegetable oil in a large skillet or wok over medium-high heat. Add tofu cubes and stir-fry until golden brown on all sides. Remove tofu from the skillet and set aside.
2. In the same skillet, add the broccoli, bell pepper, and carrot. Stir-fry for about 5 minutes until the vegetables are tender but still crisp.
3. Add the minced garlic and grated ginger, stir-frying for another minute until fragrant.

4.Return the tofu to the skillet. Add soy sauce, sesame oil, and honey. Stir well to combine all ingredients and cook for another 2 minutes.
5.Sprinkle with sesame seeds before serving.

NUTRITIONAL VALUES (PER SERVING):

✓ Calories: 350	✓ Fat: 20g	✓ Fiber: 6g
✓ Protein: 22g	✓ Carbohydrates: 24g	

PREPARATION TIPS:

• Pressing the tofu for at least 30 minutes before cooking will help it absorb more flavors and improve its texture.

SHOPPING TIPS:

• Select a variety of colorful vegetables for this dish to ensure a broad spectrum of vitamins and antioxidants.

ALTERNATIVE VARIATIONS:

• Feel free to swap out or add any vegetables you prefer, such as snap peas, mushrooms, or spinach, to customize your stir-fry.

106) EGGPLANT PARMESAN

Preparation Time: 20 minutes	**Cooking Time:** 45 minutes	**Servings:** 2

INGREDIENTS:

1 large eggplant, sliced into 1/2-inch rounds	2 eggs, beaten	1/4 cup grated Parmesan cheese
Salt	1 cup breadcrumbs	Fresh basil leaves for garnish
1/2 cup all-purpose flour	1 cup marinara sauce	
	1 cup shredded mozzarella cheese	

INSTRUCTIONS:

1.Preheat the oven to 375°F (190°C). Salt the eggplant slices and let them sit for 15 minutes to draw out moisture. Rinse and pat dry.
2.Dredge the eggplant slices in flour, dip in the beaten eggs, and then coat with breadcrumbs. Place on a baking sheet and bake for 20 minutes, flipping once, until golden.
3.In a baking dish, layer the baked eggplant with marinara sauce and mozzarella cheese, finishing with a layer of cheese on top.
4.Bake for an additional 25 minutes, or until the cheese is bubbly and golden. Sprinkle with Parmesan and fresh basil before serving.

NUTRITIONAL VALUES (PER SERVING):

✓ Calories: Approximately 600	✓ Fat: 28g	✓ Fiber: 12g
✓ Protein: 28g	✓ Carbohydrates: 62g	

PREPARATION TIPS:

• For a lighter version, grill the eggplant slices instead of breading and baking them.
• Letting the eggplant sit with salt not only draws out moisture but also reduces bitterness.

SHOPPING TIPS:

• Choose eggplants that are firm and heavy for their size, with smooth, shiny skin.
• For the breadcrumbs, consider using whole wheat for added fiber.

ALTERNATIVE VARIATIONS:

• To make this dish gluten-free, use almond flour and gluten-free breadcrumbs for the breading.
• Veganize the recipe by using plant-based cheeses and substituting the eggs with a flaxseed or chickpea flour mixture for the breading.

107) FISH TACOS WITH CABBAGE SLAW

Preparation Time: 20 minutes	**Cooking Time:** 10 minutes	**Servings:** 2

INGREDIENTS:

2 fish fillets (such as tilapia or cod)	4 small tortillas	1 tablespoon chopped cilantro
1 tablespoon olive oil	2 cups shredded cabbage	1 avocado, sliced
1 teaspoon chili powder	1/4 cup mayonnaise	Lime wedges for serving
Salt and pepper to taste	1 tablespoon lime juice	

INSTRUCTIONS:

1.Season the fish fillets with chili powder, salt, and pepper. Heat olive oil in a skillet over medium heat and cook the fish for 4-5 minutes on each side until flaky.
2.In a bowl, mix the shredded cabbage, mayonnaise, lime juice, and cilantro to make the slaw. Season with salt and pepper to taste.
3.Warm the tortillas in the oven or on a skillet.
4.Assemble the tacos by placing a piece of fish on each tortilla, topped with cabbage slaw and avocado slices.
5.Serve with lime wedges on the side.

NUTRITIONAL VALUES (PER SERVING):

✓ Calories: Approximately 500	✓ Fat: 28g	✓ Fiber: 8g
✓ Protein: 25g	✓ Carbohydrates: 44g	

PREPARATION TIPS:

• Pat the fish dry before seasoning and cooking to ensure a nice sear and prevent sticking to the pan.
• For a lighter version of the cabbage slaw, you can substitute Greek yogurt for the mayonnaise.

- When selecting fish for the tacos, look for fresh fillets that are moist, firm, and have a clean smell. If fresh isn't available, frozen fillets thawed in the refrigerator can also work well.
- For the cabbage, pre-shredded bags can save time, but shredding a whole cabbage may yield fresher results.

ALTERNATIVE VARIATIONS:

- If you're looking for a gluten-free option, use corn tortillas instead of flour ones.
- For an extra kick, add a diced jalapeño or a dash of hot sauce to the cabbage slaw.
- Vegetarians can substitute the fish with grilled or sautéed tempeh or tofu, seasoned similarly.

GARLIC LEMON BAKED SALMON

Preparation Time: 10 minutes	**Cooking Time:** 20 minutes	**Servings:** 2

INGREDIENTS:

2 salmon fillets (6 oz each)	2 garlic cloves, minced	1 tablespoon fresh dill, chopped
2 tablespoons olive oil	1 lemon, sliced	Salt and pepper to taste

INSTRUCTIONS:

1. Preheat your oven to 400°F (200°C). Line a baking sheet with parchment paper.
2. Place the salmon fillets on the baking sheet. Drizzle with olive oil and sprinkle with minced garlic, salt, and pepper.
3. Top each fillet with lemon slices and fresh dill.
4. Bake for 18-20 minutes, or until the salmon is opaque and flakes easily with a fork.
5. Serve hot, garnished with additional dill and lemon wedges on the side.

NUTRITIONAL VALUES (PER SERVING):

✓ Calories: 300	✓ Fat: 22g	✓ Fiber: 0.5g
✓ Protein: 23g	✓ Carbohydrates: 2g	

PREPARATION TIPS:

- For extra flavor, marinate the salmon in the garlic, lemon, and olive oil mixture for up to 30 minutes before baking.

SHOPPING TIPS:

- Select fresh, sustainably sourced salmon for the best taste and nutritional value.

ALTERNATIVE VARIATIONS:

- Swap salmon for trout or mackerel for a different taste while maintaining similar nutritional benefits.

108) GARLIC SHRIMP ZOODLES

Preparation Time: 15 minutes	**Cooking Time:** 10 minutes	**Servings:** 2

INGREDIENTS:

2 large zucchinis, spiralized	3 cloves garlic, minced	1 lemon, juiced
12 large shrimp, peeled and deveined	1/2 teaspoon red pepper flakes	Salt and pepper to taste
2 tablespoons olive oil	(optional)	Fresh parsley, chopped for garnish

INSTRUCTIONS:

1. Heat olive oil in a large skillet over medium heat. Add minced garlic and red pepper flakes, sautéing until fragrant.
2. Add the shrimp to the skillet and cook until they are pink and opaque, about 2-3 minutes per side. Remove shrimp from the skillet and set aside.
3. In the same skillet, add the spiralized zucchini. Sauté for about 2 minutes, or until just tender. Be careful not to overcook.
4. Return the shrimp to the skillet with the zucchini noodles. Add lemon juice and toss everything together. Season with salt and pepper to taste.
5. Serve hot, garnished with fresh parsley.

NUTRITIONAL VALUES (PER SERVING):

✓ Calories: 250	✓ Fat: 14g	✓ Fiber: 2g
✓ Protein: 24g	✓ Carbohydrates: 8g	

PREPARATION TIPS:

- Spiralize the zucchini ahead of time and store it in the refrigerator for a quick dinner assembly.

SHOPPING TIPS:

- Select zucchinis that are firm and have a vibrant green color for the best taste and texture.

ALTERNATIVE VARIATIONS:

- Add cherry tomatoes or capers to the dish for an additional layer of flavor.
- For a non-seafood version, substitute shrimp with grilled chicken strips.

109) GRILLED SALMON WITH ASPARAGUS

Preparation Time: 10 minutes	**Cooking Time:** 15 minutes	**Servings:** 2

INGREDIENTS:

2 salmon fillets (6 ounces each)	2 tablespoons olive oil	Lemon wedges for serving
1 bunch asparagus, trimmed	Salt and pepper to taste	

1. Preheat your grill to medium-high heat. Brush the salmon fillets and asparagus with olive oil and season with salt and pepper.
2. Grill the salmon, skin-side down, for 6-8 minutes. Flip and cook for an additional 4-6 minutes, or until desired doneness.
3. Grill the asparagus alongside the salmon for about 5-7 minutes, turning occasionally, until tender and charred.
4. Serve the grilled salmon and asparagus with fresh lemon wedges on the side.

NUTRITIONAL VALUES (PER SERVING):

✓ Calories: Approximately 400	✓ Fat: 28g	✓ Fiber: 3g
✓ Protein: 34g	✓ Carbohydrates: 6g	

PREPARATION TIPS:

- Letting the salmon rest at room temperature for about 10 minutes before grilling can help ensure more even cooking.
- Drizzle the asparagus with a bit of balsamic vinegar before grilling for added flavor.

SHOPPING TIPS:

- Look for fresh, sustainably sourced salmon for the best quality and flavor.
- Choose asparagus spears that are firm and bright green, with tightly closed tips.

ALTERNATIVE VARIATIONS:

- Swap asparagus for another seasonal vegetable like zucchini or bell peppers for variety.
- For a non-seafood option, grilled chicken breasts can be substituted for salmon.

110) GRILLED VEGETABLE PLATTER WITH HERBED YOGURT SAUCE

Preparation Time: 15 minutes	**Cooking Time:** 15 minutes	**Servings:** 2

INGREDIENTS:

1 zucchini, sliced lengthwise	Salt and pepper to taste	2 tablespoons chopped fresh herbs
1 yellow squash, sliced lengthwise	***For the Herbed Yogurt Sauce:***	(such as dill, parsley, and mint)
1 red bell pepper, cut into wide strips	1 cup Greek yogurt	Salt and pepper to taste
1 eggplant, sliced into rounds	2 tablespoons fresh lemon juice	
2 tablespoons olive oil	1 garlic clove, minced	

INSTRUCTIONS:

1. Preheat the grill to medium-high heat. Brush the vegetables with olive oil and season with salt and pepper.
2. Grill the vegetables in batches, turning once, until tender and charred, about 3-4 minutes per side.
3. For the sauce, combine Greek yogurt, lemon juice, minced garlic, fresh herbs, salt, and pepper in a bowl. Adjust the seasoning as needed.
4. Arrange the grilled vegetables on a platter and serve with the herbed yogurt sauce on the side.

NUTRITIONAL VALUES (PER SERVING):

✓ Calories: Approximately 280	✓ Fat: 14g	✓ Fiber: 9g
✓ Protein: 10g	✓ Carbohydrates: 34g	

PREPARATION TIPS:

- Cutting the vegetables uniformly ensures they cook evenly on the grill.
- To prevent sticking, make sure the grill is clean and well-oiled before adding the vegetables.

SHOPPING TIPS:

- Choose fresh, firm vegetables without blemishes. The fresher the produce, the better the flavor once grilled.
- For the yogurt sauce, opt for full-fat Greek yogurt for its creaminess and tang.

ALTERNATIVE VARIATIONS:

- Mix up the vegetables based on what's in season or your preferences. Asparagus, tomatoes on the vine, and corn also grill beautifully.
- For a dairy-free version of the sauce, use a plant-based yogurt and adjust the consistency with a bit of olive oil if necessary.

111) LEMON GARLIC ROASTED CHICKEN THIGHS

Preparation Time: 10 minutes	**Cooking Time:** 40 minutes	**Servings:** 2

INGREDIENTS:

4 chicken thighs, bone-in, and skin-on	4 garlic cloves, minced	1 teaspoon dried thyme
2 tablespoons olive oil	1 lemon, half juiced, and half sliced	Salt and pepper to taste

INSTRUCTIONS:

1. Preheat your oven to 400°F (200°C).
2. In a small bowl, mix olive oil, minced garlic, lemon juice, thyme, salt, and pepper.
3. Place chicken thighs on a baking sheet. Rub the olive oil mixture thoroughly over and under the skin of each thigh.
4. Arrange lemon slices around and under the chicken thighs.
5. Roast in the preheated oven for 35-40 minutes, or until the chicken skin is crispy and a meat thermometer inserted into the thickest part reads 165°F (74°C).
6. Serve hot, garnished with additional fresh thyme or parsley if desired.

NUTRITIONAL VALUES (PER SERVING):

✓ Calories: Approximately 500	✓ Fat: 36g	✓ Fiber: 0.5g
✓ Protein: 37g	✓ Carbohydrates: 4g	

PREPARATION TIPS:

• Patting the chicken dry with paper towels before applying the olive oil mixture helps achieve crispier skin.

• Letting the chicken rest for 5 minutes after roasting allows the juices to redistribute, making the meat more tender and flavorful.

SHOPPING TIPS:

• Look for chicken thighs that are similar in size to ensure even cooking.

• Fresh garlic and quality olive oil will enhance the flavor of the marinade significantly.

ALTERNATIVE VARIATIONS:

• Add root vegetables like carrots, potatoes, or parsnips around the chicken before roasting for a complete one-pan meal.

• For a spicier kick, include a pinch of red pepper flakes in the olive oil mixture.

112)   LEMON HERB ROASTED CHICKEN

Preparation Time: 10 minutes	**Cooking Time:** 45 minutes	**Servings:** 2

INGREDIENTS:

2 chicken breasts (bone-in, skin-on)	2 garlic cloves, minced	Salt and pepper to taste
1 lemon, sliced	1 teaspoon rosemary, chopped	
2 tablespoons olive oil	1 teaspoon thyme, chopped	

INSTRUCTIONS:

1. Preheat the oven to 375°F (190°C).
2. In a small bowl, mix olive oil, garlic, rosemary, thyme, salt, and pepper.
3. Rub the herb mixture all over the chicken breasts. Place the lemon slices under and on top of the chicken.
4. Roast in the preheated oven for 45 minutes, or until the chicken is cooked through and the skin is golden and crisp.
5. Let the chicken rest for 5 minutes before serving to allow the juices to redistribute.

NUTRITIONAL VALUES (PER SERVING):

✓ Calories: Approximately 400	✓ Fat: 27g	✓ Fiber: 1g
✓ Protein: 35g	✓ Carbohydrates: 4g	

PREPARATION TIPS:

• Letting the chicken rest at room temperature for about 20 minutes before cooking can help ensure more even roasting.

• For extra flavor, stuff some of the lemon slices and herbs under the skin of the chicken breasts.

SHOPPING TIPS:

• Select chicken breasts that are similar in size to ensure they cook evenly.

• When possible, choose organic or free-range chicken for the best quality and flavor.

ALTERNATIVE VARIATIONS:

• Swap chicken breasts for thighs or drumsticks if preferred; adjust cooking time accordingly.

• Experiment with different herbs like sage or parsley to create your flavor profile.

113)   LEMON HERB ROASTED TOFU WITH ASPARAGUS

Preparation Time: 15 minutes	**Cooking Time:** 25 minutes	**Servings:** 2

INGREDIENTS:

14 oz block of firm tofu, pressed and cubed	2 tablespoons olive oil	1 teaspoon dried thyme
2 cups asparagus, trimmed	1 lemon, juiced and zested	1 teaspoon dried rosemary
	2 cloves garlic, minced	Salt and pepper to taste

INSTRUCTIONS:

1. Preheat the oven to 400°F (200°C). Line a baking sheet with parchment paper.
2. In a bowl, mix olive oil, lemon juice and zest, garlic, thyme, rosemary, salt, and pepper. Add tofu cubes and asparagus, tossing gently to coat.
3. Spread the tofu and asparagus in a single layer on the prepared baking sheet.
4. Roast for 25 minutes, or until the tofu is golden and the asparagus is tender.
5. Serve hot, garnished with additional lemon zest if desired.

NUTRITIONAL VALUES (PER SERVING):

✓ Calories: 280	✓ Fat: 20g	✓ Fiber: 4g
✓ Protein: 18g	✓ Carbohydrates: 12g	

PREPARATION TIPS:

• Pressing the tofu for at least 30 minutes before marinating will ensure it absorbs more flavor.

SHOPPING TIPS:

• Select firm or extra-firm tofu for best results in texture. Look for asparagus stalks that are firm and bright green.

- For a spicy kick, add a pinch of red pepper flakes to the marinade. Swap asparagus with broccoli or green beans depending on the season.

114) LENTIL SOUP WITH KALE

Preparation Time: 15 minutes	Cooking Time: 45 minutes	Servings: 2

INGREDIENTS:

1 cup green or brown lentils, rinsed	2 stalks celery, diced	1/2 teaspoon smoked paprika
2 tablespoons olive oil	2 cloves garlic, minced	Salt and pepper to taste
1 onion, chopped	4 cups vegetable broth	2 cups chopped kale
2 carrots, diced	1 teaspoon ground cumin	Lemon wedges for serving

INSTRUCTIONS:

1. Heat olive oil in a large pot over medium heat. Add onion, carrots, and celery, cooking until softened, about 5 minutes.
2. Stir in garlic, cumin, and smoked paprika, cooking for an additional minute until fragrant.
3. Add lentils and vegetable broth. Bring to a boil, then reduce heat and simmer, covered, for about 30 minutes or until lentils are tender.
4. Stir in kale and cook until wilted about 5 minutes. Season with salt and pepper to taste.
5. Serve the soup hot, with lemon wedges on the side for squeezing.

NUTRITIONAL VALUES (PER SERVING):

✓ Calories: Approximately 400	✓ Fat: 10g	✓ Fiber: 15g
✓ Protein: 18g	✓ Carbohydrates: 60g	

PREPARATION TIPS:

- Soaking lentils beforehand can reduce cooking time and make them easier to digest.
- Adding the kale towards the end of cooking preserves its color and nutrients.

SHOPPING TIPS:

- Choose firm, dark green kale leaves for the best flavor and nutrient content.
- Lentils are available in most grocery stores; green or brown varieties hold their shape well in soups.

ALTERNATIVE VARIATIONS:

- For a heartier soup, add diced potatoes or sweet potatoes with the lentils.
- Swap kale for spinach or chard, adjusting the cooking time as these greens wilt more quickly.

115) MEDITERRANEAN STUFFED PEPPERS

Preparation Time: 20 minutes	Cooking Time: 30 minutes	Servings: 2

INGREDIENTS:

2 large bell peppers, halved and seeded	1/4 cup red onion, finely chopped	2 cloves garlic, minced
1 cup cooked quinoa	1/4 cup feta cheese, crumbled	1 teaspoon dried oregano
1/2 cup cherry tomatoes, halved	1 tablespoon olive oil, plus more for drizzling	Salt and pepper to taste
1/4 cup Kalamata olives, chopped		

INSTRUCTIONS:

1. Preheat the oven to 375°F (190°C). Place the bell pepper halves in a baking dish, drizzle with olive oil, and season with salt and pepper.
2. In a bowl, combine the cooked quinoa, cherry tomatoes, Kalamata olives, red onion, feta cheese, olive oil, garlic, oregano, salt, and pepper.
3. Stuff the quinoa mixture into each bell pepper half. Cover the baking dish with foil.
4. Bake for about 30 minutes, or until the peppers are tender.
5. Serve warm, garnished with additional feta cheese if desired.

NUTRITIONAL VALUES (PER SERVING):

✓ Calories: 360	✓ Fat: 18g	✓ Fiber: 7g
✓ Protein: 10g	✓ Carbohydrates: 42g	

PREPARATION TIPS:

- To ensure the peppers are perfectly tender, check them with a fork towards the end of baking time.
- Adjust the time as needed.

SHOPPING TIPS:

- Select firm, brightly colored bell peppers for the best flavor and presentation.

ALTERNATIVE VARIATIONS:

- For a protein boost, add chickpeas or diced chicken breast to the quinoa mixture.

116) MUSHROOM RISOTTO

Preparation Time: 10 minutes	Cooking Time: 25 minutes	Servings: 2

1 cup Arborio rice 2 tablespoons olive oil 1 small onion, finely chopped 2 garlic cloves, minced	1/2-pound mushrooms, sliced (a mix of varieties works well) 4 cups vegetable broth, warmed 1/2 cup dry white wine (optional)	Salt and pepper to taste 1/4 cup grated Parmesan cheese Fresh parsley, chopped, for garnish

INSTRUCTIONS:

1. In a large pan, heat olive oil over medium heat. Add onion and garlic, sautéing until soft and translucent.
2. Add the mushrooms and cook until they've released their moisture and begun to brown.
3. Stir in the Arborio rice, coating it in the oil and toasting slightly until the edges become translucent.
4. Pour in the white wine (if using) and stir until mostly absorbed.
5. Add the warm vegetable broth, one ladle at a time, stirring continuously until each addition is absorbed before adding the next. Continue until the rice is creamy and al dente, about 18-20 minutes.
6. Season with salt and pepper, then stir in the grated Parmesan cheese.
7. Serve the risotto garnished with fresh parsley and additional Parmesan if desired.

NUTRITIONAL VALUES (PER SERVING):

✓ Calories: Approximately 450 ✓ Protein: 12g	✓ Fat: 14g ✓ Carbohydrates: 68g	✓ Fiber: 3g

PREPARATION TIPS:

- Constant stirring is key to releasing the rice's starches, which gives risotto its creamy texture.
- For an umami boost, consider adding a splash of soy sauce or a spoonful of miso paste to the mushrooms as they cook.

SHOPPING TIPS:

- Arborio rice is essential for authentic risotto due to its high starch content. It can typically be found in the rice or international foods aisle.
- Select fresh, firm mushrooms for the best flavor. Mixing varieties like buttons, cremini, and shiitake can enhance the dish's depth.

ALTERNATIVE VARIATIONS:

- For a vegan version, omit the Parmesan cheese or use a plant-based alternative and ensure the wine is vegan-friendly.
- Add cooked chicken or shrimp to the risotto for a protein-packed meal.

117) PESTO PASTA WITH CHERRY TOMATOES

Preparation Time: 10 minutes	**Cooking Time:** 15 minutes	**Servings:** 2

INGREDIENTS:

8 oz pasta (such as penne, spaghetti, or linguine) 1 cup cherry tomatoes, halved	1/2 cup homemade or store-bought pesto Salt and pepper to taste	Grated Parmesan cheese, for serving Fresh basil leaves, for garnish

INSTRUCTIONS:

1. Cook pasta according to package instructions in a large pot of salted boiling water until al dente. Drain and return to the pot.
2. While the pasta cooks, lightly sauté the cherry tomatoes in a pan with a drizzle of olive oil over medium heat until they start to soften, about 3-4 minutes.
3. Toss the cooked pasta with the pesto until evenly coated. Gently fold in the sautéed cherry tomatoes. Season with salt and pepper to taste.
4. Serve the pesto pasta warm, topped with grated Parmesan cheese, and garnished with fresh basil leaves.

NUTRITIONAL VALUES (PER SERVING):

✓ Calories: Approximately 600 ✓ Protein: 18g	✓ Fat: 24g ✓ Carbohydrates: 80g	✓ Fiber: 5g

PREPARATION TIPS:

- To keep the pesto green and vibrant, mix it with the pasta while it's still warm but not piping hot.
- Adding a spoonful of pasta cooking water to the pesto can help create a smoother sauce that coats the pasta more evenly.

SHOPPING TIPS:

- For the freshest flavor, consider making your pesto with fresh basil, pine nuts, Parmesan cheese, garlic, and olive oil.
- When choosing cherry tomatoes, look for brightly colored, firm ones with smooth skins.

ALTERNATIVE VARIATIONS:

- For a protein boost, add grilled chicken strips or shrimp to the pasta.
- Incorporate additional vegetables like spinach, arugula, or asparagus for extra nutrients and textures.

118) QUINOA STUFFED BELL PEPPERS

Preparation Time: 20 minutes	**Cooking Time:** 30 minutes	**Servings:** 2

INGREDIENTS:

2 large bell peppers, halved and seeded 1/2 cup quinoa, rinsed	1 cup vegetable broth 1 tablespoon olive oil	1 small onion, diced 2 cloves garlic, minced

| 1/2 cup diced tomatoes
1/2 cup black beans, rinsed and
drained | 1/2 teaspoon cumin
1/2 teaspoon paprika
Salt and pepper to taste | 1/4 cup shredded cheese (optional)
Fresh cilantro for garnish |

INSTRUCTIONS:

1. Preheat the oven to 375°F (190°C).
2. In a saucepan, bring the vegetable broth to a boil. Add quinoa, cover, and simmer for 15 minutes, or until all the liquid is absorbed.
3. While the quinoa cooks, heat olive oil in a skillet over medium heat. Sauté onion and garlic until softened. Add diced tomatoes, black beans, cumin, paprika, salt, and pepper. Cook for 5 minutes.
4. Mix the cooked quinoa into the skillet with the vegetable mixture.
5. Stuff the halved bell peppers with the quinoa mixture. Place in a baking dish and cover with foil.
6. Bake for 25 minutes. Remove foil, top with cheese if using, and bake for an additional 5 minutes until the cheese is melted and the peppers are tender.
7. Garnish with fresh cilantro before serving.

NUTRITIONAL VALUES (PER SERVING):

| ✓ Calories: Approximately 320
✓ Protein: 12g | ✓ Fat: 10g
✓ Carbohydrates: 48g | ✓ Fiber: 9g |

PREPARATION TIPS:

- For a firmer pepper, reduce the initial baking time. For softer peppers, increase it.
- Adding a splash of lime juice to the quinoa mixture can enhance the flavors.

SHOPPING TIPS:

- Select bell peppers that are large and have a flat bottom, so they stand up easily in the baking dish.
- Look for quinoa in the bulk bins or grain aisle of your grocery store; it often comes in different colors, all of which are nutritious.

ALTERNATIVE VARIATIONS:

- Make it a non-vegetarian dish by adding ground turkey or beef to the quinoa mixture.
- For a vegan option, skip the cheese or use a dairy-free cheese alternative.

119)   ROASTED BUTTERNUT SQUASH SOUP

| **Preparation Time:** 15 minutes | **Cooking Time:** 45 minutes | **Servings:** 2 |

INGREDIENTS:

| 1 medium butternut squash, peeled,
seeded, and cubed
2 tablespoons olive oil
Salt and pepper to taste | 1 small onion, diced
2 garlic cloves, minced
4 cups vegetable broth
1/2 teaspoon ground cinnamon | 1/4 teaspoon nutmeg
Fresh cream for serving (optional)
Pumpkin seeds for garnish (optional) |

INSTRUCTIONS:

1. Preheat the oven to 400°F (200°C). Toss the butternut squash cubes with 1 tablespoon of olive oil, salt, and pepper. Spread on a baking sheet and roast for 25-30 minutes until tender and slightly caramelized.
2. In a large pot, heat the remaining olive oil over medium heat. Add the diced onion and garlic, sautéing until soft and translucent.
3. Add the roasted butternut squash to the pot along with the vegetable broth, cinnamon, and nutmeg. Bring to a simmer and cook for 15 minutes.
4. Puree the soup using an immersion blender or in batches with a standard blender until smooth.
5. Serve the soup warm, drizzled with fresh cream, and sprinkled with pumpkin seeds, if desired.

NUTRITIONAL VALUES (PER SERVING):

| ✓ Calories: Approximately 250
✓ Protein: 3g | ✓ Fat: 14g
✓ Carbohydrates: 34g | ✓ Fiber: 6g |

PREPARATION TIPS:

- Roasting the butternut squash before adding it to the soup enhances its natural sweetness and depth of flavor.
- If the soup is too thick, adjust the consistency by adding a bit more vegetable broth until you reach your desired thickness.

SHOPPING TIPS:

- Choose a butternut squash that feels heavy for its size with a solid beige color and no deep cuts or bruises.
- For a richer flavor, consider using homemade vegetable broth.

ALTERNATIVE VARIATIONS:

- For a vegan version, substitute fresh cream with coconut milk for serving.
- Add a spicy kick with a dash of cayenne pepper or top with roasted chickpeas for added texture and protein.

120)   SHRIMP AND BROCCOLI STIR-FRY

| **Preparation Time:** 10 minutes | **Cooking Time:** 10 minutes | **Servings:** 2 |

INGREDIENTS:

| 8 oz shrimp, peeled and deveined
2 cups broccoli florets | 2 tablespoons soy sauce
1 tablespoon oyster sauce | 1 teaspoon sesame oil
1 garlic clove, minced |

1 teaspoon ginger, minced	1 tablespoon vegetable oil	Cooked rice, for serving

INSTRUCTIONS:

1. In a small bowl, whisk together soy sauce, oyster sauce, and sesame oil. Set aside.
2. Heat vegetable oil in a large skillet or wok over medium-high heat. Add garlic and ginger, cooking until fragrant, about 1 minute.
3. Add shrimp to the skillet, stir-frying until they turn pink and opaque, about 2-3 minutes. Remove shrimp and set aside.
4. Add broccoli to the skillet, adding a splash of water. Cover and let steam until bright green and tender, about 3-4 minutes.
5. Return shrimp to the skillet, pour in the sauce mixture, and stir to combine. Cook for another 1-2 minutes, ensuring everything is heated through and coated in sauce.
6. Serve the stir-fry over cooked rice for a complete meal.

NUTRITIONAL VALUES (PER SERVING):

✓ Calories: Approximately 250	✓ Fat: 8g	✓ Fiber: 3g
✓ Protein: 23g	✓ Carbohydrates: 18g	

PREPARATION TIPS:

- For the best texture, avoid overcooking the shrimp; they should be removed from the heat as soon as they turn pink.
- Cutting the broccoli into uniform pieces ensures even cooking.

SHOPPING TIPS:

- Fresh shrimp should smell clean, briny, and slightly sweet. If buying frozen, look for shrimp that are individually quick frozen (IQF) for the best quality.
- When buying broccoli, choose heads with tight, green florets and firm stalks.

ALTERNATIVE VARIATIONS:

- Vegetarians can substitute tofu for shrimp. Press the tofu to remove excess moisture, then cube and sauté until golden before adding to the stir-fry.
- Mix in additional vegetables like bell peppers, snap peas, or carrots for more color and nutrition.

121) SPAGHETTI SQUASH WITH TOMATO SAUCE

Preparation Time: 15 minutes	**Cooking Time:** 40 minutes	**Servings:** 2

INGREDIENTS:

1 medium spaghetti squash	1 can (14 oz) diced tomatoes	Grated Parmesan cheese, for serving (optional)
2 tablespoons olive oil	1 teaspoon Italian seasoning	
1 small onion, chopped	Salt and pepper to taste	
2 garlic cloves, minced	Fresh basil leaves, for garnish	

INSTRUCTIONS:

1. Preheat the oven to 400°F (200°C). Halve the spaghetti squash lengthwise and scoop out the seeds. Brush the cut sides with 1 tablespoon olive oil and season with salt and pepper. Place cut-side down on a baking sheet and roast until tender, about 30-40 minutes.
2. Meanwhile, heat the remaining olive oil in a saucepan over medium heat. Add onion and garlic, cooking until softened. Stir in diced tomatoes and Italian seasoning. Simmer for 20 minutes, seasoning with salt and pepper to taste.
3. Once the squash is cool enough to handle, use a fork to scrape out the flesh into strands.
4. Serve the spaghetti squash topped with tomato sauce, garnished with fresh basil, and if desired, Parmesan cheese.

NUTRITIONAL VALUES (PER SERVING):

✓ Calories: Approximately 250	✓ Fat: 14g	✓ Fiber: 6g
✓ Protein: 4g	✓ Carbohydrates: 30g	

PREPARATION TIPS:

- To make the squash easier to cut, microwave it for a few minutes to soften the skin.
- For a smoother sauce, blend the tomato mixture before simmering.

SHOPPING TIPS:

- Select a spaghetti squash that feels heavy for its size with a firm, unblemished rind.
- For the tomato sauce, using fire-roasted diced tomatoes can add a depth of flavor.

ALTERNATIVE VARIATIONS:

- Add ground meat or lentils to the tomato sauce for a protein boost.
- Incorporate olives, capers, or mushrooms into the sauce for more complexity and variety.

122) SPICY CHICKPEA STEW

Preparation Time: 10 minutes	**Cooking Time:** 20 minutes	**Servings:** 2

INGREDIENTS:

1 can (15 oz) chickpeas, drained and rinsed	2 garlic cloves, minced	1/4 teaspoon cayenne pepper (adjust to taste)
2 tablespoons olive oil	1 teaspoon ground cumin	1 can (14 oz) diced tomatoes
1 onion, diced	1/2 teaspoon smoked paprika	1 cup vegetable broth

Salt and pepper to taste
Fresh cilantro, chopped, for garnish

Cooked rice or warm naan bread for serving

INSTRUCTIONS:

1. Heat the olive oil in a large pot over medium heat. Add the onion and garlic, cooking until softened.
2. Stir in the cumin, smoked paprika, and cayenne pepper, cooking for another minute until fragrant.
3. Add the chickpeas, diced tomatoes with their juice, and vegetable broth. Season with salt and pepper.
4. Bring to a simmer and cook for about 15-20 minutes, or until the stew has thickened slightly.
5. Serve the stew garnished with fresh cilantro, alongside cooked rice, or warm naan bread.

NUTRITIONAL VALUES (PER SERVING):

✓ Calories: Approximately 380	✓ Fat: 14g	✓ Fiber: 12g
✓ Protein: 14g	✓ Carbohydrates: 54g	

PREPARATION TIPS:

- For a richer stew, mash some of the chickpeas lightly before adding them to the pot. This thickens the stew without the need for additional thickeners.
- Letting the stew sit for a few hours or overnight can enhance the flavors as they meld together.

SHOPPING TIPS:

- When purchasing canned chickpeas, look for options with no added salt or preservatives to control the sodium content of the dish.
- Choose high-quality canned tomatoes for the best flavor. Fire-roasted tomatoes can add an extra dimension to the stew.

ALTERNATIVE VARIATIONS:

- Add leafy greens such as spinach or kale at the end of cooking for added color and nutrients.
- For non-vegans, topping the stew with a dollop of yogurt or sour cream can add a creamy contrast to the spicy flavors.

123) SPINACH AND FETA STUFFED CHICKEN

Preparation Time: 20 minutes	**Cooking Time:** 25 minutes	**Servings:** 2

INGREDIENTS:

2 chicken breasts	1/2 cup feta cheese, crumbled	1/2 teaspoon dried oregano
Salt and pepper to taste	1 tablespoon olive oil	
1 cup fresh spinach, chopped	1 teaspoon garlic, minced	

INSTRUCTIONS:

1. Preheat the oven to 375°F (190°C).
2. Make a deep cut along the side of each chicken breast to create a pocket. Season inside and out with salt and pepper.
3. In a bowl, mix the spinach, feta cheese, garlic, and oregano. Stuff each chicken breast with the spinach mixture.
4. In an ovenproof skillet, heat the olive oil over medium heat. Sear the chicken on both sides until golden, about 3 minutes per side.
5. Transfer the skillet to the oven and bake for 20 minutes, or until the chicken is cooked through.

NUTRITIONAL VALUES (PER SERVING):

✓ Calories: Approximately 350	✓ Fat: 18g	✓ Fiber: 1g
✓ Protein: 40g	✓ Carbohydrates: 4g	

PREPARATION TIPS:

- Be careful not to cut through the chicken breast when creating the pocket to ensure the filling stays inside while cooking.
- Searing the chicken before baking helps to lock in moisture and create a flavorful crust.

SHOPPING TIPS:

- Look for chicken breasts that are roughly the same size to ensure even cooking.
- Fresh spinach tends to have a better flavor and texture than frozen in this recipe, but make sure it's thoroughly washed.

ALTERNATIVE VARIATIONS:

- Substitute feta cheese with goat cheese or ricotta for a different flavor profile.
- For added crunch and nutrition, mix some pine nuts or walnuts into the spinach and feta filling.

124) SPINACH AND MUSHROOM STUFFED CHICKEN BREAST

Preparation Time: 20 minutes	**Cooking Time:** 25 minutes	**Servings:** 2

INGREDIENTS:

2 chicken breasts, butterfly cut	1 garlic clove, minced	Salt and pepper to taste
1 cup fresh spinach, chopped	2 tablespoons olive oil	
1/2 cup mushrooms, finely chopped	1/4 cup grated Parmesan cheese	

INSTRUCTIONS:

1. Preheat the oven to 375°F (190°C).
2. In a skillet, heat 1 tablespoon olive oil over medium heat. Add the garlic and mushrooms, cooking until the mushrooms are soft. Add the spinach and cook until just wilted. Remove from heat and let cool slightly before stirring in the Parmesan cheese.
3. Lay the chicken breasts flat and season both sides with salt and pepper. Divide the spinach and mushroom mixture between the chicken breasts, placing it on one half of each breast. Fold the other half over the top and secure it with toothpicks.

4.In an ovenproof skillet, heat the remaining olive oil over medium heat. Sear the chicken on both sides until golden, about 3 minutes per side.
5.Transfer the skillet to the oven and bake for 20 minutes, or until the chicken is cooked through.
6.Serve hot, garnished with additional Parmesan or fresh herbs if desired.

NUTRITIONAL VALUES (PER SERVING):

| ✓ Calories: 380 | ✓ Fat: 22g | ✓ Fiber: 1g |
| ✓ Protein: 38g | ✓ Carbohydrates: 4g | |

PREPARATION TIPS:

• Stuff the chicken breasts ahead of time and refrigerate until ready to cook for an even quicker dinner option.

SHOPPING TIPS:

• Choose organic chicken breasts for the highest quality and best taste.

ALTERNATIVE VARIATIONS:

• For a dairy-free version, substitute nutritional yeast for the Parmesan cheese.

125) THAI GREEN CURRY WITH VEGETABLES

Preparation Time: 15 minutes	**Cooking Time:** 20 minutes	**Servings:** 2

INGREDIENTS:

1 tablespoon vegetable oil	1 bell pepper, sliced into thin strips	1 teaspoon sugar
2 tablespoons green curry paste	1 cup broccoli florets	1/2 lime, juiced
1 can (14 oz) coconut milk	1/2 cup snap peas	Cooked jasmine rice, for serving
1 cup vegetable broth	1 tablespoon fish sauce (or soy sauce	Fresh basil or cilantro, for garnish
1 carrot, sliced into thin rounds	for a vegan version)	

INSTRUCTIONS:

1.Heat the vegetable oil in a large skillet or wok over medium heat. Add the green curry paste and fry for 1-2 minutes until fragrant.
2.Stir in the coconut milk and vegetable broth, bringing the mixture to a simmer.
3.Add the sliced carrot, bell pepper, broccoli, and snap peas to the skillet. Cook for about 10 minutes, or until the vegetables are tender but still crisp.
4.Stir in the fish sauce (or soy sauce), sugar, and lime juice. Adjust seasoning as needed.
5.Serve the curry over cooked jasmine rice, garnished with fresh basil or cilantro.

NUTRITIONAL VALUES (PER SERVING):

| ✓ Calories: Approximately 400 | ✓ Fat: 28g | ✓ Fiber: 4g |
| ✓ Protein: 6g | ✓ Carbohydrates: 34g | |

PREPARATION TIPS:

• Adjust the amount of green curry paste according to your taste preference and the spice level of the paste.
• Adding a small amount of brown sugar balances, the spice and acidity of the curry.

SHOPPING TIPS:

• Green curry paste can be found in the international aisle of most supermarkets or at Asian grocery stores.
• Choose full-fat coconut milk for a richer and creamier curry.

ALTERNATIVE VARIATIONS:

• Add tofu, chicken, or shrimp to the curry for additional protein.
• Experiment with different vegetables based on seasonality and preference, such as eggplant, zucchini, or mushrooms.

126) TOFU STIR-FRY WITH BROCCOLI AND PEPPERS

Preparation Time: 15 minutes	**Cooking Time:** 10 minutes	**Servings:** 2

INGREDIENTS:

1 block (14 oz) firm tofu, pressed and cubed	1 tablespoon vegetable oil	2 garlic cloves, minced
2 tablespoons soy sauce	1 broccoli head, cut into florets	1 tablespoon ginger, minced
1 tablespoon sesame oil	1 red bell pepper, sliced	2 tablespoons hoisin sauce
	1 yellow bell pepper, sliced	Sesame seeds for garnish

INSTRUCTIONS:

1.Marinate tofu cubes in soy sauce for at least 10 minutes.
2.Heat sesame and vegetable oils in a large skillet or wok over medium-high heat. Add marinated tofu and cook until all sides are golden brown. Remove tofu and set aside.
3.In the same skillet, add broccoli and bell peppers, stir-frying until just tender but still crisp.
4.Add garlic and ginger, cooking for an additional minute until fragrant.
5.Return the tofu to the skillet. Add hoisin sauce and toss to combine all ingredients well.
6.Serve hot, garnished with sesame seeds.

NUTRITIONAL VALUES (PER SERVING):

| ✓ Calories: Approximately 350 | ✓ Protein: 20g | ✓ Fat: 22g |

✓ Carbohydrates: 20g | ✓ Fiber: 6g

- Pressing the tofu before marinating and cooking it helps to remove excess moisture, resulting in a crispier tofu.
- For the best stir-fry, prepare all ingredients before cooking as the process is quick.

SHOPPING TIPS:

- Look for firm or extra-firm tofu for this recipe, as it holds up better during stir-frying.
- When buying hoisin sauce, check the ingredients list for added preservatives or excessive sugars.

ALTERNATIVE VARIATIONS:

- Mix in other vegetables like snap peas, carrots, or mushrooms to add different textures and flavors.
- For a gluten-free version, ensure your soy sauce and hoisin sauce are gluten-free, or substitute with tamari.

127) TURKEY CHILI

Preparation Time: 10 minutes	**Cooking Time:** 40 minutes	**Servings:** 2

INGREDIENTS:

1 lb. ground turkey	1 can (14 oz) kidney beans, drained and rinsed	Salt and pepper to taste
1 tablespoon olive oil	2 tablespoons tomato paste	Shredded cheese, sour cream, and
1 onion, diced	1 tablespoon chili powder	chopped green onions for serving
2 garlic cloves, minced	1 teaspoon cumin	
1 can (14 oz) diced tomatoes		

INSTRUCTIONS:

1. Heat olive oil in a large pot over medium heat. Add the ground turkey and cook, breaking it apart with a spoon, until browned.
2. Add the diced onion and minced garlic to the pot and sauté until the onion is translucent.
3. Stir in the diced tomatoes, kidney beans, tomato paste, chili powder, cumin, salt, and pepper.
4. Bring to a simmer and cook for 30 minutes, stirring occasionally.
5. Serve the chili hot, topped with shredded cheese, a dollop of sour cream, and green onions.

NUTRITIONAL VALUES (PER SERVING):

✓ Calories: Approximately 500	✓ Fat: 20g	✓ Fiber: 10g
✓ Protein: 40g	✓ Carbohydrates: 40g	

PREPARATION TIPS:

- For a thicker chili, let it simmer uncovered for the last 10-15 minutes of cooking to reduce the liquid.
- Adding a splash of beer or coffee can deepen the chili's flavor profile.

SHOPPING TIPS:

- Ground turkey can vary in fat content; choose lean ground turkey for a healthier option.
- For the beans, feel free to use black beans or pinto beans as an alternative to kidney beans based on your preference.

ALTERNATIVE VARIATIONS:

- Make it a vegetarian chili by substituting the ground turkey with quinoa or additional beans.
- Spice it up with diced jalapeños or chipotle peppers in adobo sauce for a smoky heat.

128) VEGETABLE CURRY WITH BROWN RICE

Preparation Time: 15 minutes	**Cooking Time:** 30 minutes	**Servings:** 2

INGREDIENTS:

1 cup brown rice	1 carrot, diced	1 can (14 oz) coconut milk
2 tablespoons coconut oil	1 bell pepper, diced	Salt and pepper to taste
1 onion, diced	1 zucchini, diced	Fresh cilantro for garnish
2 cloves garlic, minced	1 cup cauliflower florets	
1 tablespoon ginger, minced	2 tablespoons curry powder	

INSTRUCTIONS:

1. Cook the brown rice according to package instructions.
2. In a large skillet, heat the coconut oil over medium heat. Add the onion, garlic, and ginger, sautéing until the onion is translucent.
3. Add the carrot, bell pepper, zucchini, and cauliflower, cooking until slightly softened.
4. Stir in the curry powder, then add the coconut milk. Simmer for 20 minutes, or until the vegetables are tender and the sauce has thickened. Season with salt and pepper.
5. Serve the vegetable curry over the cooked brown rice, garnished with fresh cilantro.

NUTRITIONAL VALUES (PER SERVING):

✓ Calories: Approximately 500	✓ Fat: 24g	✓ Fiber: 8g
✓ Protein: 10g	✓ Carbohydrates: 68g	

PREPARATION TIPS:

- Toasting the curry powder briefly before adding the coconut milk can enhance the flavors of the spices.
- Feel free to add water or vegetable broth if the curry seems too thick.

- When buying coconut milk, look for cans labeled "unsweetened" to avoid added sugars.
- Choose a variety of vegetables for the curry to maximize the nutritional content and color of the dish.

ALTERNATIVE VARIATIONS:

- Easily make this curry a protein-packed meal by adding chickpeas, lentils, or tofu.
- For a spicier curry, include a diced chili or a teaspoon of chili flakes when sautéing the onion.

129)   VEGGIE PAD THAI

Preparation Time: 20 minutes	**Cooking Time:** 10 minutes	**Servings:** 2

INGREDIENTS:

4 ounces rice noodles	1 egg, lightly beaten (optional)	1/2 teaspoon chili powder
2 tablespoons vegetable oil	***For the sauce:***	Crushed peanuts, cilantro, and lime
1 bell pepper, julienned	2 tablespoons tamarind paste	wedges for garnish
1 carrot, julienned	2 tablespoons fish sauce (or soy sauce	
1/2 cup bean sprouts	for a vegetarian version)	
2 green onions, chopped	1 tablespoon sugar	

INSTRUCTIONS:

1. Cook rice noodles according to package instructions, then drain and set aside.
2. In a small bowl, whisk together the tamarind paste, fish sauce, sugar, and chili powder to make the sauce.
3. Heat oil in a large skillet or wok over medium-high heat. Add bell pepper and carrot, stir-frying until just tender.
4. Move the vegetables to the side of the skillet and add the egg, scrambling until just set.
5. Add the cooked noodles and sauce to the skillet, tossing everything together until well coated and heated through.
6. Stir in bean sprouts and green onions, cooking for an additional minute.
7. Serve hot, garnished with crushed peanuts, cilantro, and lime wedges on the side.

NUTRITIONAL VALUES (PER SERVING):

✓ Calories: Approximately 400	✓ Fat: 14g	✓ Fiber: 4g
✓ Protein: 10g	✓ Carbohydrates: 60g	

PREPARATION TIPS:

- Soak rice noodles in hot water instead of boiling them to prevent them from becoming too soft.
- Tamarind paste can be adjusted according to taste; start with less and add more as needed.

SHOPPING TIPS:

- Tamarind paste and fish sauce are key ingredients for authentic Pad Thai flavor and can be found in the Asian section of most supermarkets.
- Choose fresh, crisp vegetables for the best texture and flavor in your Pad Thai.

ALTERNATIVE VARIATIONS:

- Add tofu or tempeh for a protein boost. If using, pan-fry until golden before adding to the Pad Thai.
- For extra heat, serve with sriracha sauce or sliced fresh chili peppers.

130)   ZUCCHINI NOODLES WITH PESTO

Preparation Time: 15 minutes	**Cooking Time:** 0 minutes	**Servings:** 2

INGREDIENTS:

2 large zucchinis	1/4 cup pine nuts	Salt and pepper to taste
1/2 cup fresh basil leaves	2 garlic cloves	
1/4 cup grated Parmesan cheese	1/4 cup olive oil	

INSTRUCTIONS:

1. Use a spiralizer to turn the zucchini into noodles. Set aside in a large bowl.
2. In a food processor, blend basil leaves, Parmesan cheese, pine nuts, and garlic cloves. Gradually add olive oil until the mixture becomes a smooth pesto.
3. Toss the zucchini noodles with the pesto until evenly coated. Season with salt and pepper to taste.
4. Serve immediately, garnished with additional Parmesan cheese and a few basil leaves.

NUTRITIONAL VALUES (PER SERVING):

✓ Calories: Approximately 350	✓ Fat: 32g	✓ Fiber: 2g
✓ Protein: 8g	✓ Carbohydrates: 8g	

PREPARATION TIPS:

- For a crunchier texture, lightly sauté the zucchini noodles in a pan with a bit of olive oil for 1-2 minutes before tossing with pesto.
- If the pesto is too thick, add a little water or more olive oil to reach the desired consistency.

SHOPPING TIPS:

- Choose firm, medium-sized zucchini for the best noodles.
- Fresh basil leaves will give the pesto a vibrant color and flavor; however, you can substitute with spinach or kale for a different twist.

- Add cherry tomatoes, olives, or grilled chicken strips to the zoodles for extra color, texture, and protein.
- For a nut-free version of pesto, substitute sunflower seeds or hemp seeds for pine nuts.

Chapter 11.

Measurement Conversion Chart

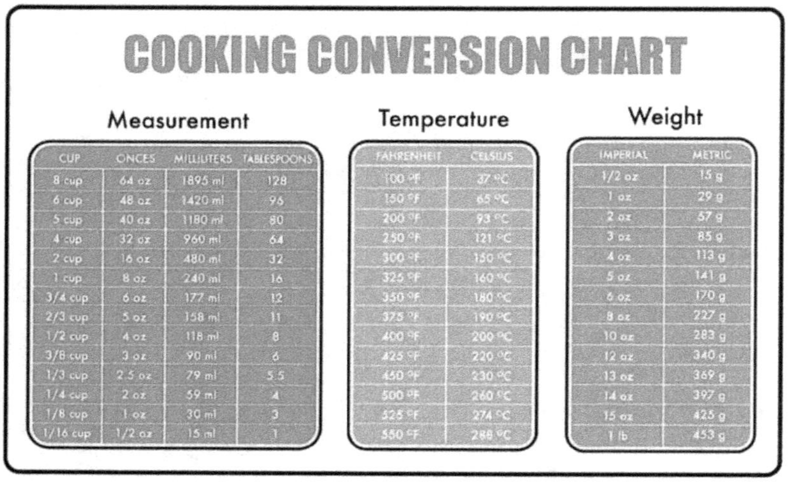

COOKING CONVERSION CHART

Measurement

CUP	ONCES	MILLILITERS	TABLESPOONS
8 cup	64 oz	1895 ml	128
6 cup	48 oz	1420 ml	96
5 cup	40 oz	1180 ml	80
4 cup	32 oz	960 ml	64
2 cup	16 oz	480 ml	32
1 cup	8 oz	240 ml	16
3/4 cup	6 oz	177 ml	12
2/3 cup	5 oz	158 ml	11
1/2 cup	4 oz	118 ml	8
3/8 cup	3 oz	90 ml	6
1/3 cup	2.5 oz	79 ml	5.5
1/4 cup	2 oz	59 ml	4
1/8 cup	1 oz	30 ml	3
1/16 cup	1/2 oz	15 ml	1

Temperature

FAHRENHEIT	CELSIUS
100 °F	37 °C
150 °F	65 °C
200 °F	93 °C
250 °F	121 °C
300 °F	150 °C
325 °F	160 °C
350 °F	180 °C
375 °F	190 °C
400 °F	200 °C
425 °F	220 °C
450 °F	230 °C
500 °F	260 °C
525 °F	274 °C
550 °F	288 °C

Weight

IMPERIAL	METRIC
1/2 oz	15 g
1 oz	29 g
2 oz	57 g
3 oz	85 g
4 oz	113 g
5 oz	141 g
6 oz	170 g
8 oz	227 g
10 oz	283 g
12 oz	340 g
13 oz	369 g
14 oz	397 g
15 oz	425 g
1 lb	453 g

11.1 Weights

Solids

g	kg	oz	lb.
30g	0.03kg	1oz	
90g	0.09kg	3oz	
125g	0.125kg	4oz	¼ lb.
250g	0.25kg	8oz	½ lb.
500g	0.5kg	16oz	1 lb.
1,000g	1kg	32oz	2 lb.
1,500g	1.5kg	48oz	3 lb.
2,000g	2 kg	64 oz	4 lb.

Liquids

Imperial measures	ml	fl oz
¼ tsp	1.25ml	
½ tsp	2.5ml	
1 tsp	5ml	⅙ fl oz
1 tsp	10ml	¼ fl oz
½ tbs	10ml	¼ fl oz
1 tbs	20ml	½ fl oz
¼ cup	60ml	2 fl oz
⅓ cup	80ml	
½ cup	125ml	4 fl oz
1 cup	250ml	8 fl oz

Ingredient	Amount	gr
Almond meal	1 cup	120gr
Almonds	1 cup	140gr
Barley, pearled uncooked	1 cup	200gr
Black beans, dry	1 cup	190gr
Breadcrumbs, dry	1 cup	90gr
Buckwheat, uncooked	1 cup	190gr
Cashews	1 cup	140gr
Chia seeds	1 tsp	5gr
Chia seeds	¼ cup	50gr
Chickpea dry	1 cup	190gr
Chickpea flour	½ cup	60gr
Cocoa powder	1 cup	100gr
Coconut, desiccated	1 cup	85gr
Couscous, uncooked	1 cup	180gr
Dates. pitted	1 cup	155gr
Flour, buckwheat	1 cup	140gr
Flour, plain	1 cup	150gr
Flour, rice	1 cup	180gr
Honey	½ cup	160gr
Kidney beans, red, dry	1 cup	190gr
Lentils, brown, dry	1 cup	210gr
Lentils, puy, dry	1 cup	200gr
Lentils, red, split, dry	1 cup	190gr
Linseeds, whole	1 tbs	5gr
Linseeds, whole	¼ cup	45gr
Milk	1 cup	250gr
Millet, hulled, uncooked	1 cup	190gr
Olive oil	1 tbs	20gr
Peanut butter	1 tbs	20gr
Peanut butter	¼ cup	70gr
Pepitas	¼ cup	40gr
Popcorn kernels	1 cup	225gr
Quinoa, uncooked	1 cup	190gr
Rice, arborio rice, uncooked	1 cup	220gr
Rice, long-grain, basmati, uncooked	1 cup	210gr
Rice, long-grain, brown, uncooked	1 cup	210gr
Rice, sushi rice, uncooked	1 cup	225gr
Rolled oats, traditional	1 cup	105gr
Sugar, raw	1 cup	205gr
Sugar, caster	1 cup	215gr
Sugar, brown	1 cup	200gr

Ingredient	Amount	gr
Sultanas	1 cup	170gr
Sunflower seeds	¼ cup	40gr
Yogurt	1 cup	250gr
Tahini	1 tbs	20gr
Tahini	¼ cup	65grr
Walnuts, whole pieces	1 cup	110gr

11.3 BAKING MEASUREMENTS

If a recipe calls for this amount	You can also measure it this way
Dash	2 or 3 drops (liquid) or less than 1/8 teaspoon of (dry)
One tablespoon of	3 teaspoons or Half ounce
Two tablespoons of	1 ounce
A quarter cup of	4 tablespoons or 2 ounces
1/3 cup	5 tablespoons plus one teaspoon
Half cup of	8 tablespoons or 4 ounces
3/4 cup	Two tablespoons of or 6 ounces
One cup of	16 tablespoons or 8 ounces
1 pint	2 cups or 16 ounces or 1 pound
1 quart	Four cups of or 2 pints
1 gallon	4 quarts
1 pound	1 ounce

11.4 VOLUME MEASUREMENTS

US Units	Canadian Units	Australian Units
A quarter teaspoon of	1 ml	1 ml
Half teaspoon of	2 ml	2 ml
One teaspoon of	5 ml	5 ml
One tablespoon of	15 ml	20 ml
A quarter cup of	50 ml	60 ml
1/3 cup	75 ml	80 ml
Half cup of	125 ml	125 ml
2/3 cup	150 ml	170 ml
3/4 cup	175 ml	190 ml
One cup of	250 ml	250 ml
1 quart	1 litre	1 litre
1 and a half quarts	One and a half litres	One and a half litres
2 quarts	2 litres	2 litres
2 and a half quarts	2.5 litres	2.5 litres
3 quarts	3 litres	3 litres
4 quarts	4 litres	4 litres

US Units	Canadian Metric	Australian Metric
1 ounce	30 grams	30 grams
2 ounces	55 grams	60 grams
3 ounces	85 grams	90 grams
4 ounces (1/4 pound)	115 grams	125 grams
8 ounces (half a pound)	225 grams	225 grams
16 ounces (1 pound)	455 grams	500 grams (half a Kg)

Fahrenheit (F)	Celsius (C) Approximate
212	100
250	120
275	140
300	150
325	160
350	180
375	190
400	200
425	220
450	230
475	240
500	260

C	F	
110°	225°	very cool
120°	250°	
140°	275°	cool
150°	300°	
160°	325°	warm
180°	350°	moderate
190°	375°	moderately hot
200°	400°	
220°	425°	
230°	450°	hot
240°	475°	very hot
250°	500°	

<u>GET YOUR EXCLUSIVE</u>
<u>BONUS NOW!</u>

Intermittent Fasting (IF) has emerged as a formidable trend in global health and fitness, widely recognized for its ability to aid in weight loss, boost overall health, and streamline dietary practices. Backed by extensive research, IF demonstrates considerable benefits not only for physical health but also for cognitive functions, with the potential to extend life expectancy. At its core, IF is distinguished by its emphasis on when to eat rather than what to eat. Popular methods such as the 16/8 and 5:2 diets provide flexible frameworks suited to diverse lifestyles and preferences. The 16/8 method confines eating to an eight-hour window each day, promoting prolonged fasting periods that are manageable and effective. Conversely, the 5:2 method allows normal eating for five days, while limiting calorie intake on two non-consecutive days to about 500–600 calories each, catering to those who may find daily fasting challenging. Empirical studies validate the effectiveness of IF in promoting significant weight loss and enhancing metabolic health. This approach capitalizes on the body's natural fasting state to burn stored fat more efficiently, thereby improving blood sugar regulation, enhancing cardiovascular health, and reducing inflammation. Such metabolic benefits underscore IF's role in not only managing but potentially reversing certain health conditions. Individuals interested in IF must consult with healthcare professionals to customize their fasting regimen according to specific health conditions and dietary needs.

This step is vital, especially to navigate potential risks associated with extended fasting periods exceeding 24 hours, which could pose health threats if not properly managed. While IF is beneficial, it is not universally suitable. Groups, especially women, might encounter varied effects due to physiological differences affecting hormones, fertility, and bone density. Consequently, IF regimens should be meticulously tailored to accommodate these specific needs, ensuring that the diet supports comprehensive health benefits without adverse effects. As with any dietary strategy, IF is often surrounded by myths and misconceptions that can deter its correct implementation. It is essential to dispel such myths to ensure safe and effective fasting practices. Contrary to common misconceptions, IF does not inherently lead to disordered eating or nutritional deficits. Proper understanding and application of IF can foster a healthy relationship with food, enhancing overall dietary satisfaction and effectiveness. The efficacy of Intermittent Fasting can significantly differ between genders, with some reports suggesting that women may experience distinct outcomes, particularly in terms of hormonal balance, fertility, and metabolic health. These differences highlight the necessity for a customized approach to fasting, ensuring that everyone's unique physiological requirements are met. For newcomers to Intermittent Fasting, such as mothers or women exploring this dietary strategy for the first time, beginning gradually is essential. The adjustment to a new eating pattern can take two to four weeks, during which feelings of hunger or irritability are common. However, those who persist through these initial challenges often find they can more easily maintain the regimen over time, experiencing sustained benefits such as weight loss, increased energy, and reduced cravings. Despite its numerous health benefits, Intermittent Fasting is often surrounded by myths and misinformation. Contrary to some claims, fasting does not inherently cause muscle loss or a significant metabolic slowdown; these misconceptions are typically rooted in outdated beliefs or misinterpretations of the fasting process. It is crucial to remain well-hydrated and nourished during eating windows to prevent adverse effects. With proper education and a deep understanding of IF principles, individuals can implement fasting safely and effectively, maximizing health benefits while minimizing risks.

Historically, fasting has been integral to human survival and cultural practices, reflecting its deep roots in our physiological makeup. In contemporary times, many are drawn to IF not only for its simplicity and direct health benefits but also to reconnect with these ancient practices. However, approaching IF with a clear understanding of its potential impacts is vital, especially for women who may need to adjust fasting durations and frequencies to accommodate their specific health needs. Intermittent Fasting has proven to be a valuable approach to nutrition, extending well beyond mere weight loss to include significant improvements in metabolic health, longevity, and disease prevention. Yet, it is not a one-size-fits-all solution; personalization and careful consideration of individual health conditions are paramount. Throughout this book, we have explored the multifaceted aspects of IF, providing a comprehensive guide to adopting this lifestyle in a manner that is informed, safe, and tailored to individual needs.

As we conclude this discussion, it is important to remember that the journey to better health through IF should be both thoughtful and informed, blending historical wisdom with modern scientific insights to achieve optimal outcomes. Whether you are just beginning your journey or seeking to refine your fasting practice, the key is to listen to your body, consult with health professionals, and make educated decisions that enhance your overall well-being. Embrace IF as a transformative tool in your health arsenal, one that promises not just a diet change, but a lifestyle evolution towards better health and longevity.